The clinical neuropsychiatry of

multiple sclerosis

This book provides a detailed survey of the emotional, behavioural and cognitive disorders prevalent among patients with multiple sclerosis (MS), including depression, mania, psychosis, pathological laughing and crying, and dementia. Attention has tended to focus on the physical aspects of MS, the commonest source of neurological disability in young and middle-aged adults, but recognition and treament of the behavioural changes associated with the disease can be equally important in improving quality of life for the patient.

For each of the neuropsychiatric disorders associated with MS, clear clinical guidelines are given for diagnosis and treatment, there is a detailed review of the literature, and case vignettes are incorporated. There are chapters on screening for cognitive deficits and neuroimaging correlates of behavioural change, and a final chapter examines the broader concept of subcortical white matter dementia. This book will be of interest to psychiatrists, neurologists, psychologists, nurses and other professionals involved in the management of patients with MS.

Anthony Feinstein is an Associate Professor in the Department of Psychiatry at the University of Toronto. He is co-director of the Traumatic Brain Injury Clinic at Sunnybrook Hospital Toronto and consultant to the MS Clinic at St Michael's Hospital Toronto.

The clinical neuropsychiatry of

multiple sclerosis

A. Feinstein, MPhil, PhD, MRCPsych, FRCP(C)

Sunnybrook Health Science Centre,
University of Toronto, Canada

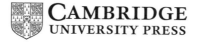
CAMBRIDGE
UNIVERSITY PRESS

PUBLISHED BY THE PRESS SYNDICATE OF THE UNIVERSITY OF CAMBRIDGE
The Pitt Building, Trumpington Street, Cambridge, United Kingdom

CAMBRIDGE UNIVERSITY PRESS
The Edinburgh Building, Cambridge CB2 2RU, UK   http://www.cup.cam.ac.uk
40 West 20th Street, New York, NY 10011-4211, USA   http://www.cup.org
10 Stamford Road, Oakleigh, Melbourne 3166, Australia

First published 1999

Printed in the United Kingdom at the University Press, Cambridge

Typeset in Minion 10/12 [VN]

A catalogue record for this book is available from the British Library

Library of Congress Cataloguing in Publication data

Feinstein, A. (Anthony), 1956–
    The clinical neuropsychiatry of multiple sclerosis / A. Feinstein.
        p.   cm.
    Includes index.
    ISBN 0 521 57274 6
    1. Multiple sclerosis – Complications.   2. Multiple sclerosis – Patients – Mental health.
    3. Psychological manifestation of general diseases.   I. Title.
    [DNLM: 1. Multiple Sclerosis – psychology.   2. Multiple Sclerosis – complications.
    3. Mental Disorders – etiology.   WL 360 f299C 1999]
    RC377.F45   1999
    616.8'34–dc21   98–46888   CIP
    DNLM/DLC
    for Library of Congress

ISBN 0 521 57274 6 hardback

To my parents

Contents

Acknowledgements

I would like to acknowledge the help of my colleagues at the University of Toronto who gave of their time and expertise. They include: at Sunnybrook Hospital, Dr Gordon Cheung (Neuroradiology), Dr Sandra Black (Behavioural Neurology) and Conrad Rockel (Research Neuroimaging); at the Baycrest Hospital, Dr Brian Levine (Neuropsychology); at St Michael's Hospital, Dr Paul O'Connor (Neurology) and Jeff Sumner (Laboratory Medicine).

Professor Maria Ron at the National Hospital for Neurology and Neurosurgery, Queen's Square, London was instrumental in first stimulating my interest in the subject of neuropsychiatric abnormalities in multiple sclerosis. Her suggestions for this book together with those from Dr Richard Barling and Joe Mottershead at the Cambridge University Press combined wisdom with perspicacity and were much appreciated.

My thanks to Sunnybrook Studios for the illustrations, Sunnybrook Medical Library staff for their assistance with some of the more obscure references and Bonnie Fabian for her secretarial skills.

Professor Ken Shulman, Chief of Psychiatry at Sunnybrook Hospital created the work environment that allowed me to write this book. Karen and Pippa, Saul and Clara, did the same on the home front.

Over the past decade, I have observed, studied and treated many patients with multiple sclerosis. The courage with which they face adversity and their commitment to demanding research protocols have been an inspiration for me.

Multiple sclerosis: diagnosis and definitions

Many a chapter, monograph and paper on multiple sclerosis begins with the observation that MS is the commonest disabling neurological disease affecting young and middle-aged adults. Since the first clinical description of the disease in the late 1830s, attention has largely focused on neurological manifestations and it is only over the past decade that clinicians, researchers, and indeed the patients themselves, have become more aware of the behavioural changes that may accompany MS. A burgeoning literature devoted to the neuropsychiatry of MS attests to this new-found interest, although those with knowledge of the medical history of MS may find themselves a little perplexed as to why it has taken so long for this interest to ignite. Descriptions of altered mentation in MS patients predate the writings of the man first credited with naming the condition over a century ago, the French behavioural neurologist Jean-Martin Charcot (Stenager, 1991).

Before describing the psychiatric and cognitive changes associated with MS, reference will be made to the neurology and pathology of the disorder. This chapter therefore begins with a summary of the pathogenesis, pathology, signs and symptoms, diagnosis and differential diagnosis of multiple sclerosis. With the book's emphasis on mentation, this introduction will by design be brief and those seeking more detailed explanations are encouraged to consult the many texts specifically devoted to these aspects. This chapter will, however, discuss in depth the research guidelines for diagnosing MS and furnish clear definitions for terms that apply directly to the disease. These points are important, for they will clarify at the outset many descriptive terms that appear in the MS research literature and are used throughout this book. The chapter will conclude with a discussion on rating disability and how behavioural changes may affect this assessment.

Epidemiology

In the United Kingdom the lifetime risk is 1:800, which translates into approximately 60 000 people with the disease (Compston, 1990). In the United States, the figure is at least four times that. There is a recognition that some cases of MS go undetected in life, appearing as a chance finding at postmortem (Gilbert and Sadler, 1983). Estimates that up to 20% of cases fall into this category (Mackay and Hirano, 1967), introduces a cautionary note in interpreting the epidemiological data. Generally, MS is seen with greater frequency as the distance from the equator increases in either hemisphere (Gonzalez-Scarano et al., 1986; Skegg et al., 1987). It is twice as common in women as in men and, although may occur at any age, onset in early adult life is commonest. The etiology is unknown, and both genetic and environmental influences are considered important. The 25% monozygotic concordance rate (Ebers and Bulman, 1986) attests to the former, while evidence of environmental influences comes from three main sources. Migration studies have demonstrated that those who emigrate during childhood assume the risk of the country of adoption (Dean, 1967), disease epidemics have been reported in isolated communities such as the Faroe Islands (Kurtzke and Hyllested, 1979), and marked variations in prevalence have been found in genetically homogeneous populations (Miller et al., 1990).

Clinical features

The disorder may present with diverse neurological signs that vary considerably between patients. Initial symptoms, which reflect the presence and distribution of the plaques, commonly involve numbness or tingling in the limbs or weakness affecting one or more limbs, loss of vision or impaired visual acuity, diplopia, facial numbness, vertigo, dysathria, ataxia and urinary frequency or urgency and fatigue. As MS is predominantly a white matter disease, symptoms referrable to cortical (grey) matter involvement are considered rare. Thus, dementia, aphasia, seizures, pain, abnormal and involuntary movement, muscle atrophy and fasciculations although possible, are so unusual they may cast doubt on the diagnosis (Rolak, 1996). The course of the disease is variable and initially impossible to predict. Approximately 5–10% of patients show a steady progression of disability from the onset of the disease. The remainder run a relapsing–remitting course, of which 20–30% never become seriously disabled and continue to function productively 20–25 years after symptom onset (Sibley, 1990). However, the largest group (almost 60%) enter a phase of progressive deterioration a variable number of years after symptom onset. Even within this group there is considerable variability, with a patient's condition fluctuating between relapses, periods of stability and progressive deterioration.

Pathology

Although the exact pathogenesis of MS is uncertain, there is firm evidence of an autoimmune mediated inflammatory disorder affecting the central nervous system (Lisak, 1986; ffrench-Constant, 1994). The target of the inflammatory response is myelin, a lipoprotein made by oligodendrocytes and investing the axons. Along the length of a nerve, the myelin sheaths are separated by gaps, the nodes of Ranvier. Nerve transmission is facilitated by impulses jumping from node to node in a process known as saltatory conduction. With damage to the myelin (i.e. demyelination), the conduction becomes impaired, transmission of nerve impulses is delayed and symptoms ensue.

Postmortem findings have further elucidated the neuropathological changes that occur (Allen, 1991). In patients severely affected by MS and who come to autopsy, the brain shows a mild degree of generalized atrophy with sulcal widening and dilatation of the ventricles. Plaques, which show histological evidence of demyelination, have a striking predilection for a bilateral periventricular distribution, particularly the lateral angles of the lateral ventricles, the floor of the aqueduct and the fourth ventricle. While plaques may also be scattered throughout the white matter, immediate subcortical myelin is usually spared and the cortex only rarely involved. When viewed on sagittal section, the relationship of demyelination to the terminal veins may be seen. In some patients, the cerebrum is relatively spared, the main lesion load involving the optic nerves, brain stem and spinal cord (Allen, 1991). Such a constellation of plaques has major implications for the presence and nature of behavioural and cognitive changes and will be more fully discussed in Chapters 2 and 9.

What exactly occurs in the early stages of demyelination is unclear, and it is the subject of debate whether demyelination can occur de novo without an observed immune response and increased cellularity, e.g. an influx of lymphocytes associated with perivascular inflammation. In the early stages of myelin breakdown, oligodendrocytes are still recognizable. As disease progresses, the myelin becomes progressively attenuated, partially detached from the axon, and ultimately phagocytozed by invading macrophages. The early, established lesion shows a characteristic pattern of increased cells (macrophages, astrocytes), a mixture of intact and disintegrated myelin sheaths, perivascular inflammation (lymphocytes, plasma cells, macrophages), oligodendrocyte loss, preserved axons, and within the grey matter, preservation of cell bodies.

In non-acute, but active plaques there is hyperplasia of macrophages and astrocytes and lesions contain myelin lipid degradation products. Perivascular inflammation, although present, is sparse. While the edges of active lesions are hypercellular with evidence of normal and disintegrating myelin sheaths, the core of such lesions may resemble older, inactive plaques. As the lesion evolves from an active to non-active phase, signs of inflammation disappear. Chronic lesions, which generally make up the bulk of the large characteristic periventricular lesions seen on MRI or at post-mortem, are thus hypocellular, demyelinated, gliosed and contain few oligodendrocytes. The demyelinated axons are separated by a heavy concentration of astrocytic processes (ffrench-Constant, 1994). The small venules are not inflamed, as in acute lesions, but rather show thickened hyalinized walls (Allen, 1991). Although considered a disease primarily affecting myelin, there is evidence that axons denuded of myelin are also susceptible to damage (Paty, 1997).

Irrespective of the stage of the lesion, remyelination may affect the changes observed. Remyelination has been noted in acute MS lesions (Prineas et al., 1993), giving rise to thin myelin sheaths in areas previously noted to be free of myelin. Newly formed as opposed to surviving oligodendrocytes are thought to be the source (Prineas et al., 1989). In chronic lesions where not all the myelin is lost, demyelination and remyelination are thought to be occurring simultaneously. In MS, remyelination is not complete, perhaps because repaired areas are subject to repeated bouts of demyelination leading to either a reduction in oligodendrocyte precursors (termed 02A progenitor cells), or the creation of an environment that inhibits their migration (ffrench-Constant, 1994).

Imaging studies during an acute attack have shown leakage of contrast enhancing materials, indicative of a breakdown in the blood–brain barrier (BBB). The compromised BBB results in edema and the entry of immune mediators (i.e. antibodies), which may contribute to myelin destruction. The leakage disappears spontaneously over 4–6 weeks (Miller et al., 1988) and may be reversed temporarily by the administration of corticosteroids (Barkhof et al., 1991). Postmortem studies have confirmed that lesions visualized on magnetic resonance imaging and computerized axial tomography correspond to MS plaques (Ormerod et al., 1987). Furthermore, an in vivo study of MRI and histological parameters from six biopsy proven cases of inflammatory demyelination of the central nervous system, has shown that changes observed on MR imaging correlate with the evolving pattern of lesions, i.e. from acute to less active to chronic (Bruck et al., 1997).

An important observation is that white matter, which appears normal to the naked eye (NAWM) will, more often than not, show histological abnormalities. These include microscopic foci of demyelination, diffuse gliosis, perivascular inflammation, deposits of iron, lipofuscin and calcium and collagenization of small blood vessels (Allen, 1991). Furthermore, this evidence of a more diffuse lesion may occur in the absence of significant plaque formation. The clinical significance of these findings is that neuroimaging of the brain and spinal cord with standard sequences devised for plaque detection, may mislead the observer into thinking the normal appearing white matter was indeed normal. Alternative imaging procedures for probing these more subtle changes have been devised, namely magnetic resonance spectroscopy, and T_1 and T_2 relaxation times, and are discussed in Chapter 9.

Diagnosis

The diagnosis of multiple sclerosis (MS) carries major implications for patients and their families. Uncertainty over the future, the ability to work, earn a living and live independently are all issues that readily come to mind. It is therefore imperative for the clinician to be clear about what symptoms and signs constitute a diagnosis of MS. In addition, making an early, correct diagnosis is assuming added importance because, for the first time, the MS patient is facing a choice of treatment options.

The diagnosis of MS is essentially a clinical one and requires that a patient of an appropriate age has had at least two episodes of neurological disturbance, implicating different sites in the central white matter. A number of investigations may help the clinician establish the presence and site of white matter lesions, thereby facilitating a diagnosis. It is, however, important to realize that these investigations (neuroimaging, evoked potentials and cerebrospinal fluid electrophoresis) are not specific for multiple sclerosis and should thus be viewed only as helpful adjuncts to the clinical presentation.

From a research perspective, correctly diagnosing MS is equally important. Researchers across sites need to talk the same language and, while well-defined clinical criteria are essential, they cannot stand apart from advances in technology. A recognition of the need to bring coherence, to what may be widely divergent neurological presentations, has prompted researchers over the years to come up with a series of diagnostic guidelines. For many years those of Schumacher (1965) sufficed, but in response to improved laboratory and clinical procedures these have given way to revised criteria (Poser et al., 1983).

The Poser Committee's Recommendations

The Poser Committee that convened in Washington, DC in 1982 comprehensively reviewed historical and clinical symptomatology in MS, immunological observations, CSF tests, a variety of neurophysiological, psychophysiological and neuropsychological procedures, neuroimaging procedures (CT and MRI), and urological studies of bladder, bowel and sexual function. They concluded that revisions to existing criteria were essential in order to conduct multicentre, therapeutic trials, to compare epidemiological data, to evaluate new diagnostic procedures and to estimate disease activity (Poser et al., 1983; Poser, 1984). It was also clear to Poser and his committee that physicians differed in their use of MS-related terminology (e.g. relapse, remission, etc.), so new definitions were included with the diagnostic criteria. They are still used today. Given the pivotal place they have assumed in MS research, and because they define concepts and categories that occur throughout this book, a detailed description follows.

Definitions

Age
For research purposes, age was limited to 10–59 years in order to minimize contamination by patients suffering from other disorders. However, it is recognized that patients may present outside this range, although such occurrences are rare.

Attack (bout, episode, exacerbation, relapse)
This was defined as the occurrence of a symptom or symptoms of neurological dysfunction, with or without objective confirmation, lasting more than 24 hours. The completely subjective nature of the symptoms were stressed, although it was acknowledged that medical corroboration would strengthen the case. Individual symptoms that were transient, such as Lhermitte's sign, i.e. sudden paresthesia following neck flexion, or vertigo lasting a few seconds, were not considered evidence of an attack.

Clinical evidence of a lesion
This refers to the demonstration of abnormal signs on examination by a competent clinician. These signs are acceptable, even if no longer present, provided they were elicited and recorded earlier by an examiner.

Paraclinical evidence of a lesion
Procedures, other than the clinical examination, that can demonstrate the existence of a lesion in the CNS are termed paraclinical evidence. The lesion may or may not have produced symptoms and signs of neurological dysfunction in the past. The procedures include evoked potential studies (Fig. 1.1), neuroimaging, most notably magnetic resonance imaging (MRI) (Fig. 1.2), and expert urological assessment.

Typical of multiple sclerosis
Certain sites within the CNS are more likely to be affected by demyelination than others, with the result that symptoms related to these sites occur more frequently. Grey matter lesions producing symptoms such as aphasia, seizures and alterations in consciousness should not be considered in making the diagnosis. However, the presence of these symptoms, in the presence of a typical clinical presentation of MS, should not invalidate the diagnosis.

Remission
A definite improvement in signs, symptoms or both that have been present

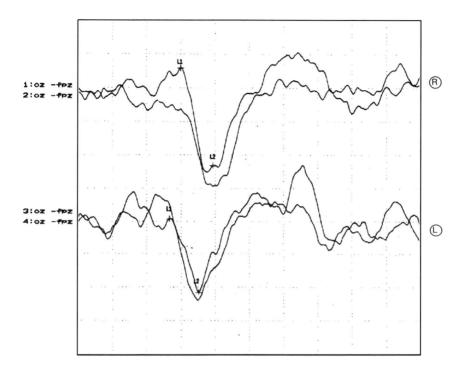

Fig. 1.1.   Visual-evoked potentials in a 33-year-old female with clinically definite MS. Note the mildly delayed conduction in the right optic nerve, compatible with optic neuritis.

for at least 24 hours is called a remission. For this to be considered clinically significant, the remission should last for a period of at least 1 month.

Separate lesions
Separate signs or symptoms cannot be accounted for by a single lesion. An example given is brainstem infarction, which may give rise to the simultaneous presentation of internuclear ophthalmoplegia, facial weakness and signs of corticospinal tract involvement. Similarly, optic neuritis affecting both eyes simultaneously is excluded. Should the second eye become involved within 15 days of the other, then convention holds that it is still regarded as a single lesion. Thus, only lesions involving distinctly different parts of the CNS satisfy the criterion.

Laboratory support
This refers only to immunological abnormalities detected in the CSF, namely increased production of immunoglobulin G (IgG) and the presence of oligoclonal bands in the absence of such bands in the serum (Fig. 1.3).

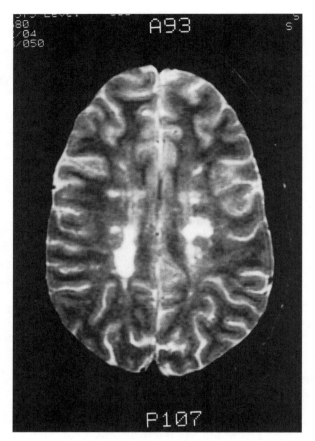

Fig. 1.2.   Axial T_2-weighted (spin echo) scan, demonstrating the extensive white matter lesions (MS plaques) in a typical periventricular distribution.

Procedures such as neuroimaging and evoked potential studies are not regarded as laboratory evidence, but rather are considered as an extension to the clinical examination (paraclinical evidence).

Associations between paraclinical and laboratory supported indices
A number of studies have investigated the degree with which the paraclinical and laboratory data are in concordance. In a study of 62 patients with clinically definite MS, Baumhefner et al. (1990) noted brain MRI abnormalities in 97% of patients, and positive oligoclonal bands in all but one of the subjects. Not all reports have yielded such strongly positive associations, however, with Pirttila and Nurmiko (1995) noting a more modest concordance rate approaching two-thirds of cases. Exploring the strength of an association between the two main paraclinical modalities, MRI abnormalities

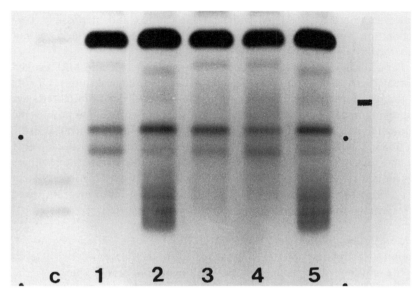

Fig. 1.3.   Abnormal oligoclonal banding in patients 2 and 5, who both have a diagnosis of laboratory supported definite multiple sclerosis.

in the brainstem have been found to correlate significantly with abnormal auditory-evoked potentials (Hendler et al., 1996), while significant correlations have also been noted between total brain MRI lesion area and delayed conduction in visual evoked potentials (Baumhefner et al., 1990).

The Poser Classification Criteria

The criteria, designed specifically for research purposes, divides MS patients into two broad groups, *definite* and *probable*, each of which may be subdivided into *clinical* and *laboratory supported*.

Clinically definite MS (CDMS)
(i)   Two attacks and clinical evidence of two separate lesions.
(ii) Two attacks; clinical evidence of one lesion and paraclinical evidence of another, separate lesion.

The two attacks must involve different parts of the central nervous system, each must last a minimum of 24 hours and be separated by a period of a month. In some cases, symptoms if considered reliable and adequate to localize a lesion typical of MS, may be accepted in lieu of clinical evidence, e.g. Lhermitte's sign in any person under 50 years of age, who does not have radiological evidence of an independent cause. Symptoms on their own must, however, only be considered with extreme caution and, if possible, corroboration from friend or relative should be sought if the attack was not recorded by a physician.

Paraclinical evidence that aids in diagnosis includes CT and MRI, evoked potentials, hyperthermia challenge and specialized urological studies. Of note is the recommendation that neuropsychological evidence of impaired cognition in someone under 50 years, although suggestive of MS, was not specific enough to be considered diagnostic. This recommendation, which was made in 1983, predated the plethora of studies from later in the decade that unequivocally demonstrated the presence of clinically significant cognitive dysfunction in approximately 40% of community-based MS patients (Rao et al., 1991a: McIntosh-Michaelis et al., 1991). To date, however, impaired cognition is still not one of the acceptable paraclinical signs.

Laboratory-supported definite MS (LSDMS)

Laboratory support comes from increased IgG in the CSF, with normal levels in the serum or oligoclonal bands in the CSF, but not in the serum.

(i)   Two attacks; either clinical or paraclinical evidence of one lesion and CSF IgG or oligoclonal bands.

(ii) One attack; clinical evidence of two separate lesions; and CSF IgG or oligoclonal bands.

(iii) One attack; clinical evidence of one lesion and paraclinical evidence of another separate lesion; CSF IgG or oligoclonal bands.

The two attacks must involve different parts of the CNS, each must last 24 hours and be separated by a month. One of the episodes must involve a part of the CNS distinct from that demonstrated by the clinical or paraclinical evidence. Unlike CDMS, historical information cannot be substituted for clinical evidence. Whether the evidence is clinical or paraclinical, both lesions must not have been present at the time of the first examination and must be separated by at least a month. This time factor is to reduce the possibility of including a case of acute disseminated encephalomyelitis.

In patients with progressive MS from symptom onset, clinical or paraclinical evidence of the second lesion should not have been present at the time of symptom onset. If the second lesion was present, the patient can only be deemed to have had MS once symptom progression had taken place for 6 months.

Clinically probable multiple sclerosis (CPMS)

(i)   Two attacks and clinical evidence of one lesion.

(ii) One attack and clinical evidence of two separate lesions.

(iii) One attack; clinical evidence of one lesion and paraclinical evidence of another separate, lesion.

The two attacks must involve separate parts of the CNS. Historical information cannot replace clinical evidence, and the restrictions discussed under *laboratory supported definite multiple sclerosis* also apply.

Laboratory supported probable multiple sclerosis (LSPMS)
(i)   Two attacks and CSF IgG or oligoclonal bands.

The two attacks must involve different parts of the CNS, must be separated by a minimum of a month and each must have lasted 24 hours.

In summary, the Poser committee acknowledge that there will always be patients who defy easy categorization. The experienced neurologist will have to rely on intuition and accumulated clinical skill in arriving at diagnoses for this group. The criteria as outlined above are primarily for research purposes. Furthermore, there is a recommendation that clinical trials and research protocols should be limited to patients in one of the two *definite* groups. The category of *probable* was designed for the purpose of prospectively evaluating new diagnostic methods.

Clinically isolated lesions

Patients with clinically isolated lesions (CIL) are of particular interest as they are frequently the forerunners of MS. In attempting to describe the natural history of psychiatric and cognitive abnormalities in MS, the study of such patients affords a valuable opportunity to document the earliest evidence of dysfunction before patients progress to the full syndrome. Throughout the book, reference will be made to patients with CIL and a brief description of these conditions is therefore given.

Optic neuritis

Acute unilateral optic neuritis (ON) in adults is the presenting feature of MS in 20% of cases, over three-quarters of patients going on to develop MS (Francis et al., 1987). It is characterized by the rapid development of visual loss, usually accompanied by pain with symptoms progressing for 3–4 weeks and then resolving over 2–3 months, recovery to 6/9 vision occurring in greater than 90% of patients (McDonald, 1983). MRI with contrast enhancement may reveal lesions within the optic nerves (Fig. 1.4). In addition, 60% of adults presenting with clinically isolated optic neuritis display one or more asymptomatic white matter brain lesions on MRI which appear indistinguishable from those seen in MS (Ormerod et al., 1987). The presence of these lesions is associated with a high risk of progression to clinically definite MS within 5 years (Miller et al., 1992), but MS should still not be diagnosed at

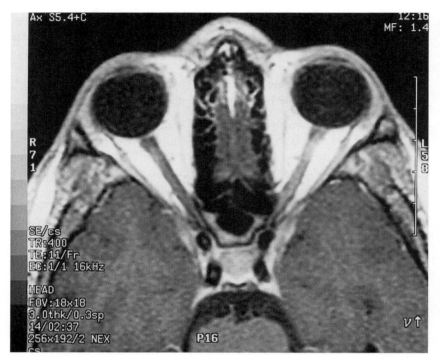

Fig. 1.4. T_1-weighted, contrast (gadolinium-DTPA)-enhanced MRI, showing pathological changes in the optic nerve in a patient with clinically definite MS.

presentation because the criterion of dissemination in space has not been satisfied.

Brainstem and spinal cord syndromes

Acute brainstem disturbance (e.g. vertigo, diplopia) is the presenting feature of MS in approximately 15% of patients, while twice as many will present with spinal cord symptoms (sensory, motor and sphincter disturbance). The percentage that go on to develop MS is probably similar to that of optic neuritis (Miller et al., 1992).

Differential diagnosis

Given the broad array and often subtle nature of neurological signs and symptoms that may herald the onset of MS, the list of conditions that make up a differential diagnosis is potentially formidable (Rolak, 1996). These include somatization disorder (hysteria), postviral demyelination (acute disseminated encephalomyelitis), vasculitis affecting the CNS (either primary or secondary conditions such as lupus erythematosus), retroviral infections such as acquired immune deficiency syndrome (AIDS), cerebrovascular accidents (stroke), metachromatic leukodystrophy and tumours (metastases, lymphoma).

To the neuropsychiatrist, dealing primarily with the behavioural sequelae of MS, the somatizing patient masquerading with MS-like symptoms can present a considerable therapeutic challenge (Aring, 1965). A follow-up of 400 patients, referred to neurologists and subsequently found not to have MS, revealed 14 with primarily psychiatric problems (Murray and Murray, 1984). These patients were more likely to be female, hospital employees or have a friend with MS and suffer from anxiety, depression and somatization disorder, the latter formerly called hysteria. Conversely, there are patients with MS, who may be incorrectly dismissed as 'hysterical'. Skegg et al. (1988) were able to identify 91 patients with MS (a point prevalence of 0.08%), of whom 16% had been referred to a psychiatrist between the onset of neurological symptoms and the diagnosis of MS. Although neurological symptoms were present at the time in the majority of patients, these had been overlooked by the psychiatrist in all but two cases. Instead, patients were given diagnoses, such as hysterical personality disorder or conversion disorder.

The clinical course of multiple sclerosis

In describing the clinical course of MS, difficulties have also been present with respect to terminology (Whitaker et al., 1995), the situation proving analogous to the imprecision that surrounded the diagnosis of MS and the definition of terms such as relapse, remission, etc. While there is general recognition that the course of MS shows individual variability, and that physical disability usually follows either a relapsing–remitting or steadily progressive course, what is meant by these terms has demanded clarification. A tightening up of terminology is not only important from a research perspective, where clear definitions of patient subgroups are essential for valid data interpretation, but also for correctly assigning patients to particular treatments. The question of which patients would benefit from which treatments is one of crucial importance to physicians looking for clear guidelines in their clinical practice.

Differences amongst researchers and clinicians in defining terms that describe the course and severity of MS have stemmed from a reliance on verbal descriptors as opposed to biological markers. This recognition led to an international survey of MS researchers, with the aim of assessing agreement pertaining to the various descriptive terms currently in use (Lublin and Reingold, 1996). The survey supplied definitions of the following disease courses and types: relapsing–remitting (RR), relapsing–progressive (RP), primary progressive (PP), secondary progressive (SP), benign and malignant. Definitions of each of these terms were included in the survey, but space was also made available for researchers to provide their own definitions if they disagreed with those enclosed. Of the 215 surveys mailed out, 125 (58%) were returned. The results led to the National Multiple Sclerosis Society (USA) providing a set of consensus definitions, which are given below.

Clinical course definitions

Relapsing–remitting (RR) MS
The consensus definition refers to clearly defined disease relapses with full recovery or with sequelae and residual deficit upon recovery; the periods between disease relapses characterized by a lack of disease progression. The defining characteristics of this course are the acute episodes of neurological deterioration with variable recovery, but a stable course between attacks (Fig. 1.5(*a*),(*b*)).

Primary–progressive (PP) MS
The consensus definition refers to disease progression from symptom onset, with occasional plateaux and temporary minor improvements allowed. The cardinal feature here is a gradual, nearly continuous worsening of neurological function from the first presentation, with some minor fluctuations but no discrete relapses (Fig. 1.6(*a*), (*b*)).

Secondary–progressive (SP) MS
This defines a course that is initially relapsing–remitting followed by a progression, with or without occasional relapses, minor remissions and plateaux. SP–MS is viewed as the long-term outcome of patients who initially show a RR–MS course. What characterizes the switch from one to the other is when the baseline between relapses begins to worsen (Fig. 1.7 (*a*), (*b*)).

Relapsing–progressive (RP) MS
There was no consensus amongst those surveyed, which was due largely to the overlap between this term and some of the other categories. The recommendation was for the term to be abandoned.

Progressive–relapsing (PR) MS
The generally agreed definition was of progressive disease from symptom onset, with clear, acute relapses, with or without full recovery; the periods between relapses were marked by continuing disease progression. PR–MS

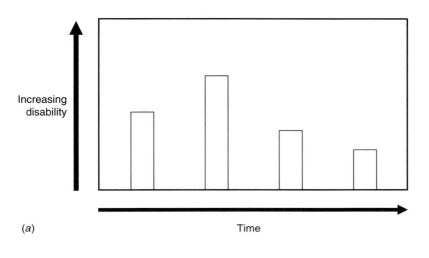

(a)   Time

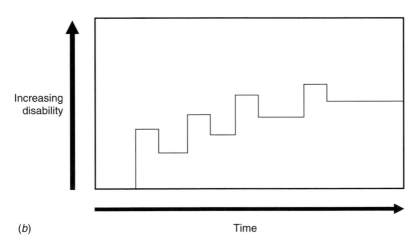

(b)   Time

Fig. 1.5.   Relapsing–remitting (RR) MS is characterized by (a) clearly defined acute attacks with full recovery (b) with sequelae and residual deficit upon recovery. Periods between disease relapses are characterized by lack of disease progression. (Lublin & Reingold, 1996). (By permission of the American Academy of Neurology.)

was considered an additional, but rare, clinical course that warranted a separate definition (Fig. 1.8 (a), (b)).

Clinical severity definitions

The merits of defining severity according to two terms, 'benign' or 'malignant' were surveyed, and the results indicated a lack of uniformity amongst

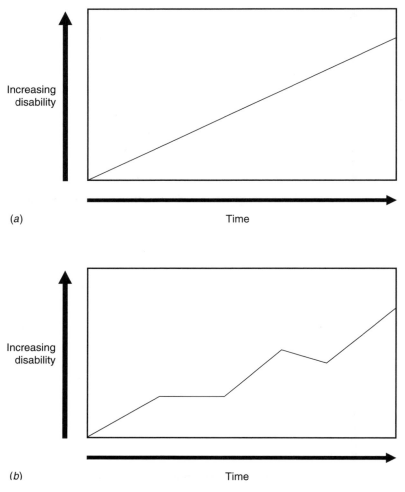

Fig. 1.6.   Primary–progressive (PP) MS is characterized by disease showing progression of disability from outset (*a*) without plateaux or remissions or (*b*) with occasional plateaux and temporary minor improvements (Lublin & Reingold, 1996). (By permission of the American Academy of Neurology.)

researchers. The disagreement was greater for what constitutes benign as opposed to malignant MS. Many respondents believed that precise definitions were not needed or useful. There was, however, agreement that the terms should not be defined according to scores on the Expanded Disability Status Scale (EDSS)(Kurtzke, 1983), the most widely used rating scale to assess physical disability in MS, as this would be too restrictive. In the end, definitions were provided with the proviso they be used primarily in a research setting.

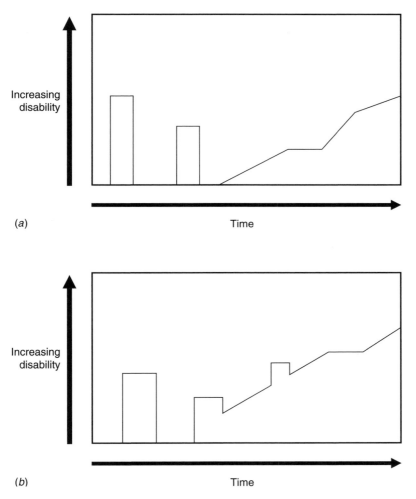

Fig. 1.7. Secondary–progressive (SP) MS begins with an initial RR course, (a) followed by progression of variable rate; (b) that may also include occasional relapses and minor remissions (Lublin & Reingold, 1996). (By permission of the American Academy of Neurology.)

Benign MS
The consensus definition was of disease in which the patient remains fully functional in all neurologic systems at least 15 years after disease onset.

Malignant MS
The consensus definition was of disease with a rapidly progressive course, leading to significant disability in multiple neurological systems or death in a relatively short time after disease onset.

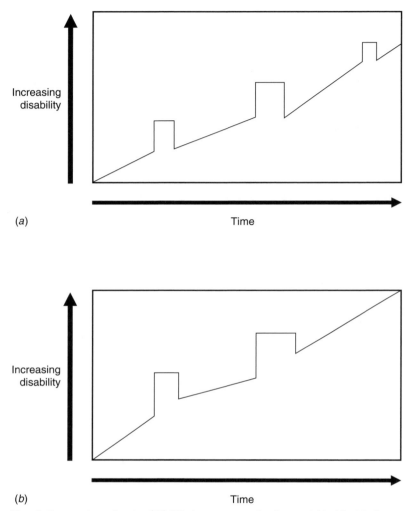

Fig. 1.8. Progressive–relapsing (PR) MS shows progression from outside (a) with clear acute relapses (b) without full recovery (Lublin & Reingold, 1996). (By permission of the American Academy of Neurology.)

In summarizing their results, Lublin and Reingold (1996) emphasized their definitions are purely clinically based and descriptive. While acknowledging the usefulness of investigations such as MRI, they concluded that current knowledge was too imprecise at this stage to allow for the course of the illness to be defined or influenced by the neuroimaging data.

In addition, the recommendations did not define what they meant by a relapse. A reason for their hesitancy in this regard was their recognition of the discordance between clinical evidence of a relapse, on the one hand, and MRI and neuropathological signs of relapse on the other. Nevertheless, the term is used repeatedly throughout their definitions, and they therefore advise that, for the purpose of a clinical trial, what is meant by relapse will need to be defined by consensus amongst investigators as part of the protocol. This view represents a clear departure from the clinical guidelines laid out by Poser et al. (1983) and illustrates a recognition that procedures such as MRI have, over the intervening 15 years, reached a level of sophistication sufficient to influence how researchers view the dynamic nature of the MS lesion.

Welcome as these guidelines are, the difficulty is assigning disease course to patients relates, in part, to the changes in neurological state that occur with time. Goodkin et al. (1989) prospectively followed a group of 254 MS patients over a 1 to 5-year-period (mean 2.6 years). They reported that adherence to the initial assigned disease course varied considerably. Thus, 30% of patients with chronic–progressive disease had become stable, 32% with stable disease had become chronic–progressive, 20% of relapsing–remitting patients had stabilized, while a similar percentage had deteriorated to a chronic–progressive phase. Furthermore, patients with either stable or relapsing–remitting (44%) disease switched as frequently to a chronic–progressive phase as patients with the latter reverted to a stable or relapsing–remitting state. The former would now be called secondary progressive disease, but the study was completed before the subdivisions of primary and secondary entered the lexicon. The implications of this study are considerable for, given the dynamic nature of the disease process, they beg the question of how valid is the assignment of disease course? Patients who qualify for interferon beta-1b therapy by virtue of having relapsing–remitting MS, may in fact have had a secondary–progressive course a few months back. Are these patients any different from those relapsing–remitting patients who have not shown a similar transformation? If so, what are the implications for treatment? The answer to these conundrums are not yet known. There is, however, an awareness that the disease is seldom static. Clearly defined definitions that carry broad agreement will ensure that if, and when, change occurs, those treating and researching multiple sclerosis patients continue to speak the same language.

Rating neurological impairment in multiple sclerosis

The yardstick by which neurological disability is rated in MS patients is the Expanded Disability Status Scale (EDSS)(Kurtzke, 1983). The scale, routinely used in clinical and research settings, represents a refinement of earlier methods devised to assess physical disability in MS (Kurtzke, 1955; Kurtzke, 1970). The scale consists of eight 'functional systems (FS)', namely pyramidal, cerebellar, brainstem, sensory, bowel and bladder, visual, cerebral (or mental) and a miscellaneous category termed 'other'. Each of these

Table 1.1. Expanded Disability Status Scale (EDSS)

0	Normal neurologic exam (all grade 0 in functional systems (FS). Cerebral grade 1 acceptable.
1.0	No disability, minimal signs in one FS (i.e. grade 1 excluding cerebral grade 1)
1.5	No disability. minimal signs in more than one FS (more than one grade 1 excluding cerebral grade 1)
2.0	Minimal disability in one FS (one FS grade 2, others 0 or 1)
2.5	Minimal disability in two FS (two FS grade 2, others 0 or 1)
3.0	Moderate disability in one FS (one FS grade 3, others 0 or 1), or mild disability in three or four FS (three/four FS grade 2, others 0 or 1) though fully ambulatory
3.5	Fully ambulatory, but with moderate disability in one FS (one grade 3) and one or two FS grade 2; or two FS grade 3; or five FS grade 2 (others 0 or 1)
4.0	Fully ambulatory without aid, self-sufficient, up and about some 12 hours a day despite relatively severe disability consisting of one FS grade 4 (others 0 or 1), or combinations of lesser grades exceeding limits of previous steps. Able to walk without aid or rest some 500 metres.
4.5	Fully ambulatory without aid, up and about much of the day, able to work a full day, may otherwise have some limitation of full activity or require minimal assistance; characterized by relatively severe disability, usually consisting of one FS grade 4 (others 0 or 1) or combinations of lesser grades exceeding limits of previous steps. Able to walk without aid or rest for some 300 metres.
5.0	Ambulatory without aid or rest for about 200 metres; disability severe enough to impair full daily activities (eg. to work full day without special provisions). (Usual FS equivalents are one grade 5 alone, others 0 or 1; or combinations of lesser grades usually exceeding specifications for step 4.0.)
5.5	Ambulatory without aid or rest for about 100 metres; disability severe enough to preclude full daily activities. (Usual FS equivalents are one grade 5 alone, others 0 or 1; or combinations of lesser grades usually exceeding those for step 4.0.)
6.0	Intermittent or unilateral constant assistance (cane, crutch or brace) required to walk about 100 metres with or without resting. (Usual FS equivalents are combinations with more than two FS grade 3+.)
6.5	Constant bilateral assistance (canes, crutches or braces) required to walk about 20 metres without resting. (Usual FS equivalents are combinations with more than two FS grade 3+.)
7.0	Unable to walk beyond 5 metres even with aid, essentially restricted to wheelchair; wheels self in standard wheelchair and transfers alone; up and about in wheelchair some 12 hours a day. (Usual FS equivalents are combinations with more than one FS grade 4+; very rarely, pyramidal grade 5 alone.)
7.5	Unable to take more than a few steps; restricted to wheelchair; may need aid in transfer; wheels self, but cannot carry on in standard wheelchair a full day; may require motorized wheelchair. (Usual FS equivalents are combinations with more than one FS grade 4+.)

8.0	Essentially restricted to bed or chair or perambulated in wheelchair, but may be out of bed itself much of the day; retains many self-care functions; generally has effective use of arms. (Usual FS equivalents are combinations, generally grade 4+ in several systems.)
8.5	Essentially restricted to bed much of the day; has some effective use of arm(s); retains some self-care functions. (Usual FS equivalents are combinations, generally 4+ in several systems.)
9.0	Helpless bed patient; can communicate and eat. (Usual FS equivalents are combinations, mostly grade 4+.)
9.5	Totally helpless bed patient; unable to communicate effectively or eat/swallow. (Usual FS equivalents are combinations, almost all grade 4+.)
10	Death due to MS

Source: Kurtzke (1983).

functional systems is rated on a 0–5 or 0–6 scale, the score determined by the results of neurological examination. The one exception to this scoring is the miscellaneous system ('other') which may be given a score of 0 or 1. The complete EDSS is given in Table 1.1.

The results of the FS ratings are collapsed down to give a total score out of 10, in increments of 0.5, which is referred to as the EDSS. An EDSS score of 0 denotes a normal neurological examination. The only symptom allowed is one of mood change, with the instruction that this should not affect the total EDSS score. An EDSS of 10 signifies death. Between these two extremes, the scale rates the level of disability with a major emphasis on the patient's ability to walk. The EDSS is thus heavily weighted in favour of pyramidal tract and brain stem involvement, with relatively little emphasis on mentation, particularly mood.

This approach is not supported by the neuropsychiatric data. There are some MS patients who are significantly disabled by a mood disorder, be it depression or mania, without a grossly abnormal neurological examination. While it is possible that such cases represent two discrete, unrelated medical disorders, i.e. MS and the mood change occurring independently of one another, the fact that, in both major depression and mania, the frequency of these disorders coexisting with MS exceeds chance expectation suggests the possibility of a causal link. Furthermore, although the high prevalence, distinct phenomenology and risks associated with mood disorders in MS have been thoroughly documented (see Chapter 2), this is not recognized by the EDSS. Sole reliance on the scale as a measure of disability may therefore lead to the erroneous impression that all is well with the patient. In the process the clinician will miss one of the most treatable causes of morbidity in MS and leave the patient at risk for potentially serious self-harm attempts (Feinstein, 1997).

The situation is only slightly better with respect to cognitive dysfunction. While the functional system devoted to mentation assigns four grades to cognitive impairment, namely mild (grade 2), moderate (grade 3), marked (grade 4) and demented (grade 5), when it comes to the full EDSS, a patient with profound dementia incapable of independent living will still only score 5.0, which denotes moderate disability. In addition, mild to moderate degrees of cognitive impairment are likely to be frequently missed when it comes to the routine neurological examination (Peyser et al., 1980) and only come to light on more detailed neuropsychological testing. With the emphasis of the EDSS so firmly rooted on ambulation, it is not surprising that correlations with indices of cognitive dysfunction are either absent or at best, weak (see Chapter 6).

There is a recognition by the committees that defined the criteria for diagnosis (Poser et al., 1983) and disease course and severity (Lublin and Reingold, 1996) that, as new knowledge comes to light, particularly from advances in areas such as neuroimaging, so the criteria will need modification. A compelling case can be made that a similar commitment to flexibility should also apply to the rating of disability in MS today. The development of the EDSS predates studies that demonstrated a high prevalence of cognitive impairment in MS (Rao et al., 1991a; McIntosh-Michaelis et al., 1991) and the accompanying social dysfunction (Rao et al., 1991b). However, while identifying the deficiencies in the EDSS may be easy, providing solutions are more complex. Despite shortcomings, the EDSS represents a quick, widely used method of quantifying physical disability. Assessing cognition, and to a lesser degree mood in MS patients, is time-consuming. The development of a rapid, accurate and easy to use procedure for rating mentation is therefore one of the challenges facing MS researchers (see Chapter 8). Whether in time the EDSS is modified to reflect a greater awareness of psychological factors will be determined largely by the outcome of this research.

Summary

- When it comes to diagnosing multiple sclerosis for research purposes, the Poser criteria are used. Four categories are specified: clinically definite, clinically probable, laboratory-supported definite and laboratory-supported probable multiple sclerosis.

- The Poser committee also specified definitions for terms such as exacerbation and remission, and what constitutes clinical, paraclinical and laboratory supported evidence of a lesion in MS.

- Definitions (according to Lublin and Reingold, 1996) are also supplied for the four recognized disease courses that the demyelinating process may follow. These are relapsing–remitting, primary–progressive, secondary–progressive, and progressive–relapsing.

- The most widely used method for rating physical disability in MS remains the Expanded Disability Status Scale (EDSS).

- The EDSS is heavily biased in favour of abnormalities affecting the pyramidal, brain stem and cerebellar systems, while difficulties with mentation receive disproportionately little attention. Thus, the EDSS is an imperfect instrument for those involved in researching the neurobehavioural aspects of MS.

References

Allen IV. (1991) Pathology of multiple sclerosis. In *McAlpine's multiple sclerosis*, ed. WB Mathews, A Compston, IV Allen, CN Martyn. Churchill Livingstone: New York, Ch. 12, pp. 341–78.

Aring SD. (1965) Observations on multiple sclerosis and conversion hysteria. *Brain*, **88**, 663–74.

Barkhof F, Hommes OR, Schettens P, Valk J. (1991) Quantitative MRI changes in gadolinium-DTPA enhancement after high dose intravenous methylprednisolone in multiple sclerosis. *Neurology*, **41**, 1219–22.

Baumhefner RW, Tourtellotte WW, Syndulko K et al. (1990) Quantitative multiple sclerosis plaque assessment with magnetic resonance imaging. Its correlation with clinical parameters, evoked potentials, and intra-blood brain barrier IgG synthesis. *Archives of Neurology*, **47**, 19–26.

Bruck W, Bitsch A, Kolenda H, Bruck Y, Stiefel M, Lassman H. (1997) Inflammatory central nervous system demyelination: correlation of magnetic resonance imaging findings with lesion pathology. *Annals of Neurology*, **42**, 783–93.

Compston DAS. (1990) The dissemination of multiple sclerosis. *Journal of the Royal College of Physicians of London*, **24**, 207–18.

Dean G. (1967) Annual incidence, prevalence and mortality of multiple sclerosis in white South Africans born and in white immigrants to South Africa. *British Medical Journal*, **2**, 724–30.

Ebers CG, Bulman DE. (1986) The geography of MS reflects genetic susceptibility. *Neurology*, **36** (suppl.), 108.

Feinstein A. (1997) Multiple sclerosis, depression and suicide. Clinicians should pay more attention to psychopathology. *British Medical Journal*, **315**, 691–2.

ffrench-Constant C. (1994) Pathogenesis of multiple sclerosis. *Lancet*, **343**, 271–4.

Francis DA, Compston DAS, Batchelor JR, McDonald WI. (1987) A reassessment of the risk of multiple sclerosis developing in patients with optic neuritis after extended follow-up. *Journal of Neurology, Neurosurgery and Psychiatry*, **50**, 758–65.

Gilbert JJ, Sadler M. (1983) Unsuspected multiple sclerosis. *Archives of Neurology*, **40**,

533–6.

Gonzalez-Scarano F, Spielman RS, Nathanson N. (1986) Epidemiology of multiple sclerosis. In *Multiple Sclerosis*, ed. WI McDonald, DH Silberberg, pp. 37–55. London: Butterworths.

Goodkin DE, Hertsgaard D, Rudick RA. (1989) Exacerbation rates and adherence to disease type in a prospectively followed-up population with multiple sclerosis. Implications for clinical trials. *Archives of Neurology*, **46**, 1107–12.

Hendler T, Squires NK, Moore JK, Coyle PK. (1996) Auditory evoked potentials in multiple sclerosis: correlations with magnetic resonance imaging. *Journal of Basic and Clinical Physiology and Pharmacology*, **7**, 245–78.

Kurtzke JF. (1955) A new scale for evaluating disability in multiple sclerosis. *Neurology (Minneapolis)*, **5**, 580–3.

Kurtzke JF. (1970) Neurologic impairment in multiple sclerosis and the Disability Status Scale. *Acta Neurologica Scandinavica*, **46**, 4493–512.

Kurtzke JF. (1983) Rating neurologic impairment in multiple sclerosis: an expanded disability status scale. *Neurology (Cleveland)*, **33**, 1444–52.

Kurtzke JF, Hyllested K. (1979) Multiple sclerosis in the Faroe Islands. 1. Clinical and epidemiological features. *Annals of Neurology*, **5**, 6–21.

Lisak RP. (1986) Immunological abnormalities in multiple sclerosis. In *Multiple Sclerosis*, ed. WI McDonald, DH Silberberg, pp. 74–98. London: Butterworths.

Lublin FD, Reingold SC, for the National Multiple Sclerosis Society (USA) Advisory Committee on Clinical Trials of new agents in multiple sclerosis (1996) Defining the clinical course of multiple sclerosis: results of an international survey. *Neurology*, **46**, 907–11.

Mackay RF, Hirano A. (1967) Forms of benign multiple sclerosis. *Archives of Neurology*, **17**, 588–600.

McDonald WI. (1983) The significance of optic neuritis. *Transactions of the Ophthalmological Society of the UK*, **103**, 230–46.

McIntosh-Michaelis SA, Wilkinson SM, Diamond ID, McLellan DL, Martin JP, Spackman AJ. (1991) The prevalence of cognitive impairment in a community survey of multiple sclerosis. *British Journal of Clinical Psychology*, **30**, 333–48.

Miller DH, Rudge P, Johnson G, Kendall BE, MacManus DG, Moseley IF, McDonald WI. (1988) Serial gadolinium enhanced MRI in multiple sclerosis. *Brain*, **111**, 927–39.

Miller DH, Hammond SR, McLeod JG, Purdie G, Skegg DCG. (1990) Multiple sclerosis in Australia and New Zealand: are the determinants genetic or environmental ? *Journal of Neurology, Neurosurgery and Psychiatry*, **53**, 903–5.

Miller DH, Morrissey SP, McDonald WI. (1992) The prognostic significance of brain MRI presentation with a single clinical episode of suspected demyelination. A 5 year follow-up study. *Neurology* (suppl. 3), 427.

Murray TJ, Murray SJ. (1984) Characteristics of patients found not to have multiple sclerosis. *Canadian Medical Association Journal*, **131**, 336–7.

Ormerod IEC, Miller DH, McDonald WI et al. (1987) The role of NMR imaging in the assessment of multiple sclerosis and isolated neurological lesions. *Brain*, **110**, 1579–616.

Paty DW. (1997) MRI as a method to reveal pathology in MS. *Journal of Neural Transmission*, **49** (suppl.), 211–17.

Peyser JM, Edwards KR, Poser CM, Filskov SB. (1980) Cognitive function in patients with multiple sclerosis. *Archives of Neurology*, **37**, 577–9.

Pirttila T, Nurmiko T. (1995) CSF oligoclonal bands, MRI, and the diagnosis of multiple sclerosis. *Acta Neurologica Scandinavica*, **92**, 468–71.

Poser CM. (1984) Taxonomy and diagnostic parameters in multiple sclerosis. *Annals of the New York Academy of Sciences*, **436**, 233–45.

Poser CM, Paty DW, Scheinberg L et al. (1983) New diagnostic criteria for multiple sclerosis: guidelines for research protocols. *Annals of Neurology*, **13**, 227–31.

Prineas JW, Barnard RO, Kwon EE, Sharer LR, Cho ES. (1993) Multiple sclerosis: remyelination of nascent lesions. *Annals of Neurology*, **33**, 137–51.

Prineas JW, Kwon EE, Goldenberg PZ, Ilyas AA, Quarles RH, Benjamins JA, Sprinkle TJ. (1989) Multiple sclerosis: oligodendrocyte proliferation and differentiation in fresh lesions. *Laboratory Investigation*, **61**, 489–503.

Rao SM, Leo GJ, Bernardin L, Unverzagt F. (1991a) Cognitive dysfunction in multiple sclerosis. 1. Frequency, patterns and prediction. *Neurology*, **41**, 685–91.

Rao SM, Leo GJ, Ellington L, Nauertz T, Bernardin L, Unverzagt F. (1991b) Cognitive dysfunction in multiple sclerosis. 2. Impact on employment and social functioning. *Neurology*, **41**, 692–6.

Rolak LA. (1996) Multiple sclerosis. In *Office Practice of Neurology*, ed. MA Samuels, S Feske). pp. 350–3. New York: Churchill Livingstone.

Schumacher GA, Beebe GW, Kibler RF et al. (1965) Problems of experimental trails of therapy in multiple sclerosis. *Annals of the New York Academy of Sciences*, **122**, 552–68.

Skegg DCG, Cormin PA, Craven RS, Malloch JA, Pollock M. (1987) *Journal of Neurology, Neurosurgery and Psychiatry*, **50**, 134–9.

Skegg K, Corwin PA, Skegg DCG. (1988) How often is multiple sclerosis mistaken for a psychiatric disorder? *Psychological Medicine*, **18**, 733–6.

Sibley WA. (1990) Diagnosis and course in multiple sclerosis. In *Neurobehavioural aspects of multiple sclerosis*, ed. SM Rao, pp. 5–14. New York: Oxford University Press.

Stenager E. (1991) Historical and psychiatric aspects of multiple sclerosis. *Acta Psychiatrica Scandinavica*, 84, 398.

Whitaker JN, McFarland HF, Rudge P, Reingold SC. (1995) Outcome assessment in multiple sclerosis clinical trials: a critical analysis. *Multiple Sclerosis*, **1**, 37–47.

2

Multiple sclerosis and depression

Of all the mental state changes associated with MS, depression in various forms is by far the commonest. It is therefore important that the clinician has a good understanding of how the syndrome may present, what factors may underlie causation and how best to approach treatment. A recent review undertaken by the author of 100 consecutive MS referrals to his neuro-psychiatry clinic revealed that over 80% had mood disorders, the majority having 'major' depression. The referrals had all been made by neurologists attached to the clinic. Over half the depressed patients had already been started on antidepressant therapy by the time they were seen. The result was that most of these patients presented a lot more cheerfully to the clinic than they had done 1 month earlier to the neurologist. This is not to decry the role of the specialist neuropsychiatrist in managing depression. There will always be patients with treatment-resistant depression, or those who have difficulty tolerating medication, or those in whom the 'talking therapies' may be indicated either alone or as an adjunct to pharmacotherapy. Given that treatment offers such rewarding possibilities, a higher profile for this par-ticular aspect of MS seems overdue.

Conceptual issues

The observation that depression is frequently part of the clinical picture of MS can be traced back to the observations of Charcot (1877). The term depression is, however, often loosely applied to describe either a symptom or syndromes of varying severity, with the spectrum including transient changes in mood, adjustment disorders to life events, dysthymia and major depres-sion with or without psychotic features. The heterogenous nature of the depressive syndrome is further illustrated by the Research Diagnostic Criteria (Endicott and Spitzer, 1978, 1979) subdivision of major depression into no fewer than ten different categories, namely primary, secondary, recurrent, psychotic, incapacitating, endogenous, agitated, retarded, situational and simple, in the process adding to semantic confusion. Common to all, how-ever, is the cardinal feature of low mood.

More recently, the classification has undergone another revision, with the fourth edition of the Diagnostic and Statistical Manual (DSM-1V)(APA,

Table 2.1. DSM-1V diagnostic criteria for mood disorders due to a general medical condition

A.	A prominent and persistent disturbance in mood predominates in the clinical picture and is characterized by either (or both) of the following:
(i)	depressed mood or markedly diminished interest or pleasure in all, or almost all, activities.
(ii)	elevated, expansive, or irritable mood.
B.	There is evidence from the history, physical examination, or laboratory findings that the disturbance is the direct physiological consequences of a general medical condition.
C.	The disturbance is not better accounted for by another mental disorder (e.g. adjustment disorder with depressed mood in response to the stress of having a general medical condition).
D.	The disturbance does not occur exclusively during the course of a delirium.
E.	The symptoms cause clinically significant distress or impairment in social, occupational, or other important areas of functioning.

Specify type:

With depressive features: if the predominant mood is depressed, but the full criteria are not met for a major depressive episode.

With major depressive-like episode: if the full criteria are met (except criterion D) for a Major Depressive Episode.

With manic features: if the predominant mood is elevated, euphoric or irritable.

With mixed features: if the symptoms of both mania and depression are present, but neither predominates.

Reprinted with permission. © 1994 American Psychiatric Association.

1994) dropping the term Organic Mood Disorder and replacing it with the category 'Mood disorder due to a general medical condition', of which four subtypes are specified (Table 2.1). The criteria for a major depression are shown in Table 2.2. Omitting the word organic has been a major conceptual leap, implying that most symptoms of mental illness are attributable, in varying degrees, to cerebral pathology. While few would doubt the biological basis to mood change, one cannot always assume that when depression occurs in the context of a general medical condition, the latter is the primary etiological factor. This point is well illustrated by the relationship of depression to MS. Unlike the search for cerebral correlates of cognitive dysfunction, which has yielded many significant correlations, similar efforts with depression have been largely unsuccessful. Possible reasons for this will be reviewed, but first, the findings pertaining to prevalence, symptom constellations, depression as a presenting feature of MS, the natural history of depressive change and depression in relation to physical disability and disease duration will be discussed. The chapter concludes with a section devoted to different treatment modalities.

Table 2.2. DSM-1V criteria for a major depressive episode

A.	Five (or more) of the following symptoms have been present during the same 2–week period and represent a change from previous functioning; at least one of the symptoms is either (i) depressed mood or (ii) loss of interest or pleasure.
(i)	depressed mood most of the day, nearly every day, as indicated by either subjective report (e.g. feels sad or empty) or observation made by others (e.g. appears tearful). *Note:* in children or adolescents, can be irritable mood.
(ii)	markedly diminished interest or pleasure in all, or almost all, activities of the day, nearly every day (as indicated by either subjective account or observation made by others).
(iii)	significant weight loss when not dieting or weight gain (e.g. change of more than 5% of body weight in a month), or decrease or increase in appetite nearly every day. *Note:* in children, consider failure to make expected weight gains.
(iv)	insomnia or hypersomnia nearly every day.
(v)	psychomotor agitation or retardation nearly every day (observable by others, not merely subjective feelings of restlessness or being slowed down).
(vi)	fatigue or loss of energy nearly every day.
(vii)	feelings of worthlessness or excessive or inappropriate guilt (which may be delusional) nearly every day (not merely self-reproach or guilt about being sick).
(viii)	diminished ability to think or concentrate, or indecisiveness, nearly every day (either by subjective account or observed by others)
(ix)	recurrent thoughts of death (not just fear of dying), recurrent suicidal ideation without specific plan, or a suicide attempt or a specific plan for committing suicide.
B.	The symptoms do not meet the criteria for a mixed episode.
C.	The symptoms cause clinically significant distress or impairment in social, occupational, or other important areas of functioning.
D.	The symptoms are not due to the direct physiological effects of a substance (e.g. a drug of abuse, a medication) or a general medical condition (e.g. hypothyroidism).
E.	The symptoms are not better accounted for by bereavement, i.e. after the loss of a loved one, the symptoms persist for longer than 2 months or are characterized by marked functional impairment, morbid preoccupation with worthlessness, suicidal ideation, psychotic symptoms or psychomotor retardation.

Prevalence of depression in MS

The frequency of depressive disorders has varied according to the cohort studied and method used. In addition, some studies have looked at point and/or lifetime prevalence rates while others at prevalence figures since the onset of MS.

Conflicting evidence exists on whether there is an increase in depression prior to the onset of neurological symptoms in MS. While Whitlock and Siskind (1980) and Joffe et al. (1987a) are of the opinion there is, this has not been noted by Ron and Logsdail (1989) nor Minden et al. (1987), the latter finding that rates did not differ from those in a healthy community sample matched for age.

These figures contrast with those found in patients with established MS. A number of studies have used the lifetime version of the Schedule for Affective Disorders and Schizophrenia (SADS-L) which enables Research Diagnostic Criteria (RDC) diagnoses to be made. Minden et al. (1987) noted a 54% lifetime prevalence while Schiffer et al. (1983), in a sample of 30 cases, found a 37% prevalence of major depression since the onset of the MS. In a study of 100 consecutive attenders at an outpatient clinic, Joffe et al. (1987a) found a 47% lifetime prevalence of major depression and a 14% prevalence of current depression, with a further 13% of the sample experiencing lesser degrees of depressive illness over their lifetime. Most recently, Sadovnik et al. (1996) have reported a lifetime prevalence of DSM-111–R major depression in 50% of MS patients. The results of a meta-analysis confirm an increased prevalence of major depression in MS compared to other neurological disorders (Schubert and Foliart, 1993).

These figures are in accord with prevalence rates obtained from self-report questionnaires, of which the Beck Depression Inventory has been the most frequently used (Minden et al. 1987; Joffe et al. 1987; Beatty et al. 1988a, 1989; Ron and Logsdail, 1989), although it should be noted that such an approach is not geared towards establishing a diagnosis.

In summary, pooling figures from published reports, the lifetime prevalence for major depression due to MS, varies from 25–50% (Minden and Schiffer, 1990). This is almost three times the lifetime prevalence reported in the general population by the National co-morbidity study (Kessler et al., 1994).

The symptoms of depression

Mood change associated with MS may present in a number of ways. While the *syndrome* of major depression has been shown to have a 12–month prevalence rate of 34%, individual symptoms comprising the syndrome such as depression (64%), anger (64%), irritability (56%), and discouragement (42%) are more frequently reported (Minden et al., 1987). However, a more cautionary note should be introduced here. The heterogenous nature of the syndrome and the potential for confusing certain somatic complaints of multiple sclerosis, such as fatigue and sleeplessness, with symptoms of depression, may lead to falsely elevated prevalence rates. It is therefore advisable that, when assessing depression in MS, attention should be focused on low mood as the cardinal feature with abnormalities in 'vegetative features' considered of doubtful significance, a view endorsed by others (Nyenhuis et al., 1995).

The difficulty in disentangling somatic complaints due to MS from those attributable to depression is highlighted by the symptom of fatigue. This was one of the symptoms most frequently endorsed by patients on the Clinical Interview Schedule (Ron and Logsdail, 1989), thereby raising the question of whether it is a psychological or a physical symptom or a combination of the two. Krupp el al (1988) believe the fatigue of MS is a distinct entity unrelated to neurological impairment, affective disorder and qualitatively different from fatigue experienced by healthy individuals. Whether or not this is a valid assumption, this ubiquitous symptom is unlikely to exist in isolation and may influence other aspects of the mental state such as concentration, memory, irritability and sleep patterns and, in turn, be aggravated by low mood.

These diagnostic pitfalls have not, however, gone unnoticed. Even with the somatically loaded questions removed from rating scales such as the Beck Depression Inventory, the prevalence of depression still remains significantly elevated. Similarly, if care is taken during the clinical interview before attributing symptoms such as 'loss of enjoyment of activities' to depression as opposed to the underlying neurological disorder, the conclusions reached are the same, namely that major depression occurs significantly more often in MS than in many other neurological disorder and healthy control subjects (Minden et al., 1987).

There is also evidence to suggest that a major depressive-like disorder due to multiple sclerosis differs from uncomplicated major depression. The typical picture commonly found in the latter, i.e. withdrawn and apathetic, with feelings of guilt and worthlessness is unusual. Rather, symptoms such as irritability, worry and discouragement predominate (Minden et al., 1987). A high frequency of irritability has also been confirmed by others (Ron and Logsdail, 1989).

These points are well illustrated by the following clinical vignettes.

A 37-year-old mother of two children aged 10 and 8 years, working part-time as a secretary was referred to my neuropsychiatry clinic because of low mood. The patient had had MS for 4 years, was in a relapsing–remitting course, had an EDSS of 3.5 and had recently experienced an exacerbation from which she had made a full recovery. There was no premorbid nor family history of psychiatric illness. Although the patient complained of feeling depressed, closer questioning revealed her main difficulties were fatigue and having to look after her two young children while holding down a job. Her marriage was described as good, but her husband was frequently away from home on business trips and the running of the household was left to her. There was no history of sleep nor appetite disturbance, no suicidal thought, but some mild anhedonia, linked specifically to periods of fatigue. Significantly, the patient reported that when her parents took the grand-children for a weekend, she felt 'restored' and better able to enjoy a good book or a visit with a friend. Her problem was assessed as primarily situational rather than a mood disorder and psychosocial intervention, while only partially alleviating her fatigue, rapidly restored her mood.

A 25-year-old woman, unmarried, working as a receptionist with a 2-year history of relapsing–remitting MS and an EDSS of 4.0 presented to my clinic with complaints of tiredness, low mood and loss of emotional control. She had been sleeping poorly for approximately 1 month and was slowly withdrawing from social contacts, as she preferred being alone. There was no premorbid nor family history of psychiatric difficulties and she was known to be an outgoing and gregarious person by nature. There had been a couple of incidents at work in which she reported 'snapping' at customers over the telephone and her company had received one complaint about this. The behaviour was most uncharacteristic of her and she found it upsetting. Her boyfriend of 3 years reported similar, unprovoked outbursts. Despite taking a few weeks off work 'to sort herself out', the irritability, sleep difficulties and social withdrawal had not improved and she had begun questioning whether life was indeed worth living. A diagnosis of mood disorder due to MS (Major Depressive subtype) was made and the appropriate pharmacotherapy instituted.

Psychiatric presentations of multiple sclerosis

Although some cases of MS presenting with psychiatric symptoms (including depression) have been reported (Young et al., 1976; Mathews, 1979; Whitlock and Siskind, 1980), the evidence from epidemiological studies suggests it is uncommon and may be a chance finding. A comparison of rates of psychiatric illness in large samples of patients with MS and temporal lobe epilepsy (TLE)(Schiffer and Babigian, 1984) revealed that, although 17% of the MS group *initially* presented to a psychiatrist, this was significantly less than the 29% reported for TLE. This figure is similar to the 19% prevalence reported by Stenager and Jensen (1988), who found the onset of the disease coincided with psychotic disorders and transient situational disturbances, but not with depressive nor anxiety disorders. While both these studies make the point that psychiatric illness may predate the onset of neurological symptoms, often by years, no unequivocal conclusions can be drawn concerning a shared pathogenesis as it is possible the two disorders may have co-existed purely by chance, given that both are common. In addition, it can be notoriously difficult to accurately document retrospectively the first, often subtle neurological symptoms heralding the onset of MS, which makes the interpretation of data such as these potentially difficult.

Nevertheless, in a well-defined regional population, Skegg et al. (1988) were able to identify 91 patients with MS (a point prevalence of 0.08%) of whom 16% had been referred to a psychiatrist between the onset of their symptoms and the diagnosis of MS. Although neurological symptoms were present at the time in the majority of patients, these had been overlooked by the psychiatrists in all but two cases. Instead, patients were given diagnoses such as hysteria more often than depression.

Depression, physical disability and duration of MS

The questions of disease duration and physical disability present difficulties when it comes to drawing etiological inferences, and the facts to date have been contradictory. While Whitlock and Siskind (1980) and McIvor et al. (1984) have reported a positive association between depression and physical disability, no such relationship between depression (Minden et al., 1987) and emotional dysfunction (Rabins et al., 1986; Ron and Logsdail, 1989) on the one hand, and disease duration, severity or course on the other, has been noted.

The reason for the lack of a clear association between disease duration and psychiatric problems is likely due to the diversity in the course of MS. Thus, an illness with the same duration may involve either a few, mild relapses or follow a more malignant, rapidly progressive course. It may also encompass patients with either quiescent lesions or those with a rapidly deteriorating lesion load. Similarly, the degree of physical disability may be determined by a combination of cerebral and spinal cord involvement, each having a different influence on affect.

Etiology of depression in MS

The pathogenesis of the major depressive-like disorders, frequently experienced by MS patients, is unclear. Research looking at the genetics of mood and

MS, structural neuroimaging, endocrine dysfunction, immune system abnormalities and social variables has been completed, but no clear picture has emerged. The reasons for these partial successes and failures are reviewed and future research options suggested.

Genetics and depression

There is no evidence to suggest a genetic link between MS and unipolar depression. Based on the family history method, Joffe et al. (1987b) did not find an excess of affective illness in the first-degree relatives of patients with MS, a finding in agreement with others (Minden et al., 1987; Schiffer et al., 1988). This is in contrast to the strong familial linkage noted in patients with uncomplicated major depression (Gershon et al., 1982).

However, with respect to depression occurring as part of bipolar affective illness, the question is less clear (see section on Bipolar Affective Disorder).

Epidemiological data

Using a computer search of medical and psychiatric records in Monroe county, New York, Schiffer and Babigian (1984) found a significantly higher rate of depression in patients with MS compared to those with temporal lobe epilepsy and amyotrophic lateral sclerosis (ALS). The data with regard to ALS is particularly compelling, given the invariably poor prognosis associated with the condition and tends to suggest that depression in MS cannot be construed simply as a reaction to physical disability. This data supported the conclusions of Whitlock and Siskind (1980), who noted that MS patients experienced more depressive episodes than those with other neurological disorders, such as muscular dystrophy, motor neurone disease and dystrophica myotonia. An earlier study by Surridge (1969) comparing MS and muscular dystrophy patients had however failed to find differences in the prevalence of depression, but the study was flawed owing to an absence of standardized assessment procedures and failure to control for levels of disability.

Comparisons between MS patients and controls with spinal cord injuries

Rabins et al. (1986) noted higher scores on the 28–item General Health Questionnaire (GHQ) in MS patients with brain involvement on CT scan when compared to a control group with spinal cord injuries. Similarly, Schiffer et al. (1983) compared two groups of 15 MS patients with either predominantly brain or spinal cord involvement based on clinical assessment and CT scan findings. Despite being matched for age, duration of illness and degree of physical disability, the former had significantly more major depressive episodes.

Depression and MS exacerbations

Dalos et al. (1983) undertook a longitudinal study over the course of 1 year, assessing MS patients at monthly intervals with a self-report measure of psychological distress, namely the General Health Questionnaire (GHQ). The instrument contains four subscales measuring depression, anxiety, somatic complaints and social dysfunction. Patients with spinal cord injuries were used as controls. Higher GHQ scores with regard to social dysfunction and somatic complaints were noted in the MS sample, particularly those experiencing disease exacerbations. However, no firm conclusions about the role of cerebral pathology can be drawn from this study for a host of reasons. The failure to find differences in depression scores between MS patients (irrespective of exacerbations), and controls may have been due to the inadequacy of the GHQ in probing the phenomenology of depression in MS. Furthermore, increased GHQ scores with disease exacerbation may simply reflect a psychological reaction to deteriorating neurological status. Finally, spinal cord as opposed to brain involvement may have triggered the relapse. Fortunately, the sensitivity of MRI in detecting brain lesions in MS has the potential to clarify some of these confounding factors.

MRI studies and depression

Three studies have reported a positive association, but two are methodologically flawed. Honer et al. (1987), using direct, computerized lesion detection, compared the MRI findings in eight patients with MS and abnormal mental states with those of eight MS control patients matched for age, sex, duration and disability, but without psychiatric impairment. DSM-111 (American Psychiatric Association, 1980) diagnoses were major depression (3), bipolar affective disorder (2), organic hallucinosis (1), organic affective syndrome (1) and organic personality disorder (1). Although the two groups did not differ with respect to total lesion load, the psychiatric group had significantly more temporal lobe involvement. This study, however, suffers from a small sample size (only four patients with depressive illness) and magnetic resonance images obtained with a weak field strength (0.15 tesla), which would have compromised lesion detection and quantification. A second study with a larger sample size (Reischies et al., 1988) found that periventricular and discrete frontal lesions were associated with psychopathology, but the absence of a standardized psychiatric assessment compromises the results. A third study by Pujol et al. (1997) offers the best evidence of a link between brain pathology and depression. The authors focused specifically on frontal areas of the brain, and despite using a self-report questionnaire as the sole index of depression, noted that lesions in the left suprainsular white matter, which includes the arcuate fasciculus, accounted for a statistically significant 17% of the depression score variance.

The above findings have been offset by a greater number of studies failing to report an association between brain involvement and depression (Huber et al., 1987; Logsdail et al., 1988; Anzola et al., 1990; Ron and Logsdail, 1989; Feinstein et al., 1992a, b). Rather, a more robust association has been found between depression and MS patients' perceived levels of social stress and support (Ron and Logsdail, 1989; Feinstein et al., 1992b). Although these studies all used MRI, methodological problems meant their results have to be interpreted with caution. These limitations pertain to three areas, namely the method of psychiatric assessment, MRI scanning parameters and MRI data analysis.

Psychiatric assessment
Some studies relied on self-report questionnaires for a diagnosis of major depression (Huber et al., 1987; Anzola et al., 1990; Feinstein et al., 1992a). Such a process lacks validity and is not a substitute for in-depth mental state examination using established interview schedules. In other studies, more global evidence of psychopathology was obtained (anxiety, phobias, insomnia, depression, etc) without attention being directed specifically at major depression (Logsdail et al., 1988; Ron and Logsdail, 1989; Feinstein et al., 1992b).

MRI scanning parameters
The majority of MRI studies have followed a similar procedure, namely using T_2-weighted and/or proton density spin echo sequences, considered preferable for demonstrating the presence of MS plaques. The failure to differentiate acute from chronic lesions with contrast media such as gadolinium-diethyl triamine penta-acetic acid (DTPA) and predominantly T_1-weighted images may account for some MRI studies that have not found an association between lesion load and anatomical distribution, on the one hand, and depression on the other.

There is, however, tentative evidence from one serial MRI study, suggesting depression may be precipitated by active brain lesions (Feinstein et al., 1993). Ten patients with relapsing–remitting MS underwent contrast-enhanced MRI and psychological assessment every 2 to 4 weeks for a period of 6 months. Only two patients showed MRI evidence of active disease and, in both, worsening depression scores significantly paralleled an increase in lesion enhancement area.

MRI data analysis
Studies aimed at detecting brain lesions and quantifying their volume have used two approaches. An early and inferior method (Logsdail et al., 1988; Anzola et al., 1990; Ron and Logsdail, 1989; Feinstein et al., 1992b) relied on viewing the MRI hard copy and assigning a rating to lesion size. This method is significantly less sensitive than a more sophisticated one consisting of viewing the brain slices on a computer console and using relevant software to measure lesion area and volume (Rao et al., 1989).

In summary, evidence from imaging studies in MS linking major depression to brain involvement is, at best, equivocal. Positive associations are limited either to a single, early and relatively insensitive MRI study with a small sample size, or to an even earlier CT study using patients with spinal cord injury as controls. These findings are offset by a larger number of MRI studies failing to report an association, the results of the latter compromised by an inadequate assessment of depression, an absence of contrast enhanced scanning sequences and outmoded MRI data analysis.

Neuroimaging data in depressed MS patients contrast with those found in other neurological disorders. Thus, in stroke patients a firm association between poststroke depression and lesions situated in the anterior aspect of the left (dominant) frontal lobe (Robinson et al., 1983; Starkstein and Robinson, 1989) has been noted. It is postulated that depression results from vascular lesions disrupting the neural circuit linking the frontal cortex to the striatum, thereby interfering with biogenic amine pathways.

Functional imaging
The often diffuse nature of brain pathology in MS has not lent the condition to functional brain imaging with positron emission tomography (PET) or single photon emission computerized tomography (SPECT), and thus no study has been undertaken looking specifically at correlates of depression. However, with regard to other primarily subcortical conditions, results have been informative. A study using fluorodeoxyglucose PET found that depressed, as opposed to non-depressed, patients with Parkinson's disease had lower metabolism in the caudate nuclei and orbital frontal cortex (Mayberg et al., 1990). Similarly, depressed patients with Huntington's disease had reduced caudate, putamen, and cingulate metabolism, in addition to reductions in orbital frontal and inferior prefrontal cortical areas (Mayberg et al., 1992). The overlap with the Parkinson data led the authors to conclude that depression in both disorders was due to a selective dysfunction of paralimbic, frontal brain regions.

Other causes

Abnormalities in the hypothalamic–pituitary–adrenal (HPA) axis of patients with MS have been documented (Michelson et al., 1994; Wei and Lightman, 1997), including failure to suppress cortisol in depressed and non-depressed patients after dexamethasone administration (Reder et al., 1987). Whether these changes are etiologically implicated in depression is unclear, although a study that correlated depression with HPA axis abnormalities and contrast-enhanced brain lesions on MRI suggests they are (Fassbender et al., 1998). Similarly, although an association between depression and dysregulation of the immune system has been reported in MS patients (Foley et al., 1992), what is cause and effect is not yet known. A related, unanswered question is posed by the possible mood-altering properties of certain drugs such as interferon beta-1b (Neilley et al., 1996), recommended for the treatment of patients with relapsing–remitting MS. While prospective evidence is still awaited, treatment of depression improves adherence to therapy with the drug, pointing to the possibility of an association (Mohr et al., 1997).

From the perspective of a neuropsychiatrist, it remains hard to look beyond the lesions demonstrated by MRI. Further research, however, is needed using improved methodology, different MRI scanning parameters and contrast enhancing compounds such as gadolinium-DTPA. Notwithstanding this, social factors should not be dismissed prematurely in the search for etiology. The mean age of disease onset in MS is considerably earlier than in stroke, Parkinson's and Huntington's disease, and the difficulties faced by young patients confronting the possibility of lifelong disability, often with little hope of cure, are formidable. In bringing together disparate etiological theories, explanations like 'multifactorial' cannot be avoided. Unsatisfactory as it may seem, particularly in relation to the literature on secondary depression in other neurological disorders, it may, in fact, represent the most accurate explanation why so many patients with MS become depressed (Feinstein, 1995).

The natural history of mood change in MS

Data suggesting an absence of major depression and a low overall psychiatric morbidity early in the disease process (Logsdail et al., 1988; Feinstein et al., 1992a) have come from studies of patients with clinically isolated lesions (optic neuritis, brainstem and spinal cord presentations), frequently the harbinger of MS. Prevalence rates for emotional distress in this group did not exceed those reported from normal community samples (Andrews et al., 1977) nor general practice attenders (Goldberg and Blackwell, 1970). A study of patients with optic neuritis and MS of less than 2 years' duration reached similar conclusions (Lyon-Caen et al., 1986).

A follow-up study of patients with CIL offered Feinstein et al. (1992b) the opportunity to chart the evolution of mood change as demyelination progressed. After a period of 5 years (range 42–67 months) 54% of patients had developed clinically definite MS, 34% with a relapsing–remitting and 20% with a chronic–progressive course. Overall, psychiatric morbidity had increased with time, but was confined to patients who had developed MS. In those whose condition had remained unchanged (i.e. CIL at follow-up) mood remained euthymic. The chronic–progressive subgroup were more physically disabled and had more extensive brain plaques. Their depression scores were three times those of the CIL and relapsing-remitting MS groups, but mood correlations were found, not with brain total lesion load, but rather with social variables.

While the above study demonstrated that patients become significantly more depressed when the disease progresses from CIL to definite MS status, it did not address the question of possible fluctuations in depressed mood, over time, in patients with established MS. Of interest was the relationship between depression, on the one hand, and alterations in clinical state and brain lesion load, on the other. The interaction between these variables is complex because changes in brain MRI are not always mirrored by changes in neurological status and associated physical disability (Thompson et al., 1992). The possibility therefore existed that changes in mood and cognition were more sensitive markers of alterations in brain lesion scores than were physical signs. A longitudinal study of ten patients with relapsing–remitting MS individually matched with ten healthy control subjects provided evidence to support this (Feinstein et al., 1993). Over a 6-month period MS patients underwent MRI at either two-weekly ($n=5$) or four-weekly intervals depending on whether they were in an active or remitted disease state. At each radiological assessment, patients were assessed neurologically and completed a mood questionnaire. Two of the five patients in an active phase of the disease had increasing lesion scores. There was also an increase in the number and size of lesions that enhanced with gadolinium-DTPA, indicating disease activity. Despite the deteriorating MRI picture, there was no concomitant decline in physical disability according to scores on the Expanded Disability Status Scale (EDSS). Both patients had, however, become increasingly depressed, and their changing depression scores correlated significantly with their MRI data. The remaining patients demonstrated little disease activity on serial MRI and their EDSS and depression scores remained stable over time.

Suicide in MS

While the presence of a major depressive illness significantly increases the morbidity associated with MS, it may also add to the mortality. Kahana et al. (1971) reported that 3% of 295 patients committed suicide over a 6-year period, but it is unclear how representative the sample was or how many subjects were suffering from a depressive illness. This figure contrasts with a lifetime prevalence of approximately 1% reported for suicide attempts in a general population study, of which less than 1 in 10 would be expected to succeed (Paykel et al., 1974). More recent data tend to confirm Kahana's observations. A study of suicide in patients with a wide range of neurological disorders (Stenager and Stenager, 1992) concluded that the rate was increased in disorders such as MS and in certain subgroups of epilepsy. In addition, an epidemiological investigation confined to a sample of 5525 MS patients (Stenager et al., 1992) reported a significantly elevated suicide rate, with males and those diagnosed with MS before the age of 30 years most at risk. Once again, no precise estimates of depression were obtained, but given the close association between MS and depression, they are likely to have been high. Further epidemiological evidence of an increased mortality in MS because of suicide comes from Sadovnik et al. (1991). In a study of 3126 MS patients followed up over 16 years, suicide accounted for 15% of all ascertained deaths, which was 7.5 times that for the age, but not sex-matched general population.

Indirect evidence linking depression and suicide comes from a study that reported low nocturnal melatonin secretion in MS patients with suicidal behaviour or intent (Sandyk and Awerbach, 1993). Serotonin is a precursor to melatonin, and a reduction in serotonergic activity has been reported in MS (Johansson and Roos, 1974) and in non-MS subjects who were depressed and committed suicide (Shaw et al., 1967). The detection of the depressed patient is therefore of the utmost importance, for it represents one of the most treatable causes of morbidity and mortality in MS (Feinstein, 1997).

Having stressed the importance of failing to detect the suicidal MS patient, it is important to place these findings in perspective. Although the chances statistically of an MS patient committing suicide are increased, the actual numbers of patients who do so are very small. It is more common for patients to entertain a vague notion of self-harm, without formulating any definite plan in that regard. A survey recently conducted at the MS clinic at St Michael's Hospital in Toronto revealed that, at any one point in time, 22% of clinic attenders harboured thoughts of suicide with varying degrees of seriousness (A. Feinstein, unpublished data). However, only a small fraction of this group will ever act on the thought, and an even smaller percentage will do so successfully.

Treatment

Treatment of depression need not be the preserve of the psychiatrist. Schiffer (1987), who has characterized depressive reactions as biological, social, or psychological suggests each may respond to specific interventions well within the therapeutic skills of the attending neurologist. Should the neurologist prove unequal to the task, Schiffer wittily recommends the 'Edward V11' approach, namely abdicating authority for psychological management to those more experienced in treating psychopathology.

Medication

It is surprising that, given the frequency with which major depression occurs in MS, only a single, double blind placebo-controlled drug trial has been reported (Schiffer and Wineman, 1990). Of 28 patients with MS, 14 were randomly assigned to a 5-week trial of desipramine and individual psychotherapy, and 14 to placebo and psychotherapy. All subjects met the criteria for major depression. The mean dose of desipramine taken was 123.2± 60.8 mg per day and seven patients in the drug treatment group were unable to reach their desired serum level because of untoward side effects. These included postural hypotension, dry mouth and constipation, which were more common in the drug group, but which also occurred in the placebo-treated patients. Patients on desipramine showed a statistically significant improvement in mood compared to the placebo group, according to scores on the Hamilton rating scale. The attainment of the therapeutic window was not of crucial significance in that patients taking the drug still improved at subthreshold levels. The authors concluded that desipramine was of modest benefit to depressed patients with MS, but side effects remained a problem, limiting the dose and thereby the response.

In an open trial 11 MS patients were treated with 100 mg of sertraline, a selective serotonin reuptake inhibitor (SSRI). All ten patients who remained on treatment for at least 3 months improved and none reported side effects (Scott et al., 1995). A retrospective review tends to support the efficacy of antidepressant medication, with over 50% of patients relapsing if medication was stopped (Scott et al., 1996). The SSRI drugs were generally better tolerated than the tricyclics, although they too were not without their side effects, which included nausea, sexual dysfunction, insomnia, palpitations, tremor, and anorexia in varying combinations in 16% of patients.

The remaining reports of response to psychotropic medication have been anecdotal, but also illustrate that newer classes of antidepressant drugs such as the SSRIs are easier to tolerate and likely to be equally or more effective. Thus, Shafey (1992) reported a case of depression that did not respond to 225 mg/day of a tricyclic drug (doxepin), but returned to an euthymic state on 40 mg/day of fluoxetine. Flax et al. (1991) also noted good responses to fluoxetine in 20 patients with MS who all tolerated the drug well. The one discordant note came from Browning (1990) who documented an exacerbation in neurological symptoms in a single patient just started on fluoxetine. The significance of this one case report is difficult to assess in the absence of controlled treatment trials, but it is likely that the exacerbation was either a chance occurrence or a rare adverse drug reaction.

Until such time as double blind placebo trials are undertaken, it would therefore seem prudent to use an SSRI or selective noradrenaline reuptake inhibitor as a first choice, switching to another drug in the same class if treatment response is unsatisfactory. Adding lithium as an adjunct would be the next step if an antidepressant alone proved ineffective. There is no evidence in MS patients that any one SSRI is better than another, but the preference for fluoxetine may reflect the perception amongst clinicians that the drug is helpful with some neurological symptoms as well, particularly fatigue. Once again, this evidence is anecdotal. A practical point to follow when starting treatment is not to discontinue the drug in response to complaints such as constipation or dry mouth, but rather to reduce the dosage. Clinical experience dictates that certain patients respond better, with less severe side effects, to 10 mg as opposed to the more frequently prescribed 20 mg. The use of alternative classes of antidepressant drugs with a potentially activating profile, such as the monoamine oxidase inhibitors or buproprion, have not been evaluated, although the latter, as an adjunct in treating SSRI-induced sexual dysfunction, may prove benficial.

A 32-year-old married accountant with a 5-year history of MS and an EDSS of 3.5 presented to his family doctor with a 6-week history of low mood, irritability, some vegetative features and thoughts of suicide. Desipramine had been started and the dose gradually titrated upwards, with some improvement in mood and partial resolution of insomnia. However, at doses greater than 100 mg per day, the patient reported excessive drowsiness and a very unpleasant dry mouth and requested he come off the treatment. At this point he was referred to my clinic. The medication was discontinued over the course of a week, and 20 mg of fluoxetine was started as a replacement. A marked improvement in mood was noted within 2 weeks and the medication was well tolerated apart from erectile dysfunction, not previously reported. Reducing the dosage of fluoxetine to 10 mg did not restore sexual function, although mood remained euthymic. The patient elected to remain on the fluoxetine stating he could 'live with the (sexual) problem, but not with the depression'. However, after 6 months of normal mood he changed his mind and asked once again to come off treatment. Given the disabling nature of his depression and the earlier plans for self-harm when depressed, I was reluctant to discontinue treatment after only 6 months. The addition of 75 mg buproprion OD, an antidepressant with little seretonergic effect, brought about a resolution in the erectile difficulties.

Cognitive-behaviour therapy

In a well-controlled study, Larcombe and Wilson (1984) found cognitive-behaviour therapy (CBT) to be more effective than no treatment when it came to alleviating symptoms of depression. Sample size was small, with nine patients receiving CBT and ten patients put on a waiting list without intervention. CBT took place in groups with weekly sessions of $1\frac{1}{2}$ hours. Treatment continued for 6 weeks. All subjects had been carefully screened to ensure patients met the criteria (Feighner et al., 1972) for 'definite' or 'probable' depression and to exclude patients with cognitive dysfunction, the presence of which may have compromised therapy. At the end of the trial, the patients receiving CBT showed a significant improvement in mood as judged by four separate assessment procedures, namely a self-report scale, a clinician rating scale, a rating made by a 'significant other' (close friend, family member) and a measure of daily mood.

The efficacy of CBT in treating patients with depression of mild to moderate severity has been well documented in patients with uncomplicated depression (Rush et al., 1977; Blackburn et al., 1986) and as such, the results in the MS sample should come as little surprise. In MS patients, CBT has the advantage over medication of an absence of troubling side effects. The fact that CBT works well in groups is another advantage, for it enhances the cost-effectiveness of the procedure. It is, however, limited to cognitively intact patients, who would need to be screened prior to enrolment in a treatment group. Similarly, there would not be a place for CBT in the severely depressed, suicidal patient. Here, antidepressant medication is the treatment of choice, with the more rapid onset of action of the SSRI drugs making them the preferred option.

A variant of CBT is Stress Inoculation Training (SIT), a short-term, cognitive-behavioural approach that targets maladaptive psychological responses to stress, thereby enhancing coping mechanisms. Such a technique, in combination with progressive deep muscle relaxation, has been applied effectively to MS patients in a case control study (Foley et al., 1987).

Psychotherapy

Individual psychotherapy

An approach to psychotherapy for patients with MS has been eloquently summarized by Minden (1992). She stresses a practical, common sense approach to therapy, decrying the notion that only supportive therapy is required and debunking the myth that patients have to be 'psychologically minded' to be suitable candidates for this treatment modality. Varying degrees of psychological distress will be present at different times in the disease course because of the dynamic nature of a disease process characterized by relapses and remissions and the impossibility of predicting what the future holds. The fluctuating feelings of despair, fear, hopelessness alternating with optimism, hope and relative wellbeing demands flexibility from the therapist. During periods of disease exacerbation and psychological distress, supportive therapy intermingled with practical advice to the patient seems more appropriate than attempts at dealing with unresolved, hidden conflicts that may be well defended. Conversely, during remissions in the disease, frequently accompanied by emotional equanimity, more detailed insight-oriented psychoanalytic therapy may prove beneficial. The use of pharmacotherapy as an adjunct is not ruled out. This flexible approach extends to deciding the duration of treatment, which may vary from a single session to treatment over years, depending on the needs of the patient. Although there are no empirical data to support the efficacy of Minden's approach, the overriding emphasis on humaneness and the appeal to intuitive common sense has much to recommend it.

Group therapy

A number of early reports suggested that group therapy with MS patients was advantageous in relieving psychological distress. The approaches have been varied; psychoanalytic (Barnes et al., 1954; Day et al., 1953), supportive-analytical (Bolding, 1960), supportive (Spielberg, 1980) and a more simple, educational approach with spouses and family also involved Pavlou et al. (1979). What all these studies had in common, however, was their largely anecdotal nature, with an absence of control groups and a failure to employ pre- and post-treatment assessment measures.

Crawford and McIvor (1985) corrected many of these methodological shortcomings in their outcome study in which 41 MS patients were divided into three groups: insight-orientated psychotherapy, current events discussion and non-treatment. Patients were assessed over a 6-month period. Although the three groups were equally depressed at entry to the study, only patients receiving the insight-orientated psychotherapy showed a significantly mood improvement. Although the study illustrates the benefits of insight-orientated group psychotherapy to patients with MS, the result has not been replicated. Similarly, the efficacy of other forms of group therapy have yet to be evaluated. Applying Minden's (1992) philosophy concerning individual psychotherapy to a group setting, it seems equally plausible to believe that, when required, simple supportive therapy, in which practical advice is dispensed, questions answered and distress openly acknowledged, would prove beneficial to patients. Such a view, however, awaits empirical validation.

Electroconvulsive therapy

The use of electroconvulsive therapy (ECT) has been reported in a small number of MS patients and found to be effective (Gallineck and Kalinowsky, 1958; Krystal and Coffey, 1997), although treatment has been associated with an exacerbation in MS symptoms in approximately 20% of cases. The presence of contrast enhancing lesions on MRI prior to ECT has been identified as a possible risk factor for neurological deterioration (Mattingley et al., 1992). The high rate of complications suggests ECT should be used only if the patient has not first responded to pharmacotherapy or if the mental state was such that emergency treatment was required, e.g. the severely depressed, actively suicidal patient. Contrast-enhanced MRI may also guide the treatment decisions.

Herbal remedies

It is not uncommon for MS patients to self-medicate, and a host of preparations, available without prescription, have been tried ranging from the legal (e.g. evening oil of primrose) to the outlawed (e.g. cannabis). Depressed MS patients have resorted to St John's wort (*Hypericum perforatum*), and there is evidence from a meta-analysis that this decision has some merit. Linde et al. (1996) reviewed the data from 23 randomized clinical trials (none confined to MS patients) and concluded the herb was more effective than placebo in mild to moderately severe depression. Precisely how the medication exerts antidepressant effects is not known. Furthermore, use of St John's wort was not given an unqualified endorsement, for efficacy in comparison with SSRI or tricyclic drugs, and its use in treating more severe forms of depression, has yet to be established.

Summary

- Clinically significant depression (DSM-1V major depression) in association with MS has a lifetime prevalence of approximately 50%.
- MS patients have a significantly increased rate of suicide compared to the general population and patients with other neurological disorders. As yet, there is no study proving a link between suicide and depression, although such as association appears likely.
- MS patients do not appear to have a premorbid risk for affective disorder. Major depression in MS patients is frequently associated with irritability and a sense of frustration, as opposed to symptoms of guilt and worthlessness that are more typically found in major depression without MS.
- Unlike cognitive dysfunction, there is, as yet no clear association between

MRI demonstrated brain abnormalities and major depression. The failure of MRI studies to find such an association may relate, in large part, to methodological limitations inherent in the studies.

• There is a suggestion that immune abnormalities, in association with dysfunction of the hypothalamic–pituitary–adrenal axis, may be the mechanism underlying the high lifetime risk for major depression.

• There is only one double blind, placebo-controlled trial of antidepressant medication in depressed MS patients and this demonstrated the clinical efficacy of the tricyclic antidepressant, desipramine. Anecdotal evidence, however, points towards newer antidepressants such as the SSRI drugs as the treatment of choice, because of their less troublesome side effects.

• Psychotherapy, either individual or group, is also helpful particularly for less severe depression. In more severe cases, it may prove a useful addition to antidepressant medication.

• In patients who do not respond to antidepressant medication, lithium augmentation of the antidepressant drug may prove effective.

• ECT may be used in severe cases of drug refractory depression, although there appears to be a 20% risk of triggering a MS relapse. The presence of active brain lesions on MRI pre-ECT is a potential risk factor for neurological relapse following treatment.

• It needs to be emphasized that depression represents a considerable source of morbidity and mortality in MS, and missing the diagnosis does the patient a great disservice, more so as the disorder can, in the majority of patients, be successfully treated.

References

American Psychiatric Association. (1980) *Diagnostic and Statistical Manual of Mental Disorders*. Third Edition. American Psychiatric Association: Washington, DC.

American Psychiatric Association (1994) Diagnostic and Statistical Manual of Mental Disorders. Fourth Edition. American Psychiatric Association: Washington, DC.

Andrews G, Schonell M, Tennent C. (1977) The relationship between physical, psychological and social morbidity in a suburban community. *American Journal of Epidemiology*, **105**, 324–9.

Anzola GP, Bevilacqua L, Cappa SF et al. (1990) Neuropsychological assessment in patients with relapsing–remitting multiple sclerosis and mild functional impairment: correlation with magnetic resonance imaging. *Journal of Neurology, Neurosurgery and Psychiatry*, **53**, 142–5.

Barnes RH, Busse EW, Dinken H. (1954) Alleviation of emotional problems in multiple sclerosis by group psychotherapy. *Group Psychotherapy*, **6**, 193–201.

Beatty WW, Goodkin DE, Monson N, Beatty PA, Hertsgaard D. (1988) Anterograde and retrograde amnesia in patients with chronic–progressive multiple sclerosis. *Archives of Neurology*, **45**, 611–19.

Beatty WW, Goodkin DE, Monson N, Beatty PA. (1989) Cognitive disturbance in patients with relapsing–remitting multiple sclerosis. *Archives of Neurology*, **46**, 1113–19.

Blackburn IM, Eunson KM, Bishop S. (1986) A two-year naturalistic follow-up of depressed patients treated with cognitive therapy, pharmacotherapy and a combination of both. *Journal of Affective Disorders*, **10**, 67–75.

Bolding H. (1960) Psychotherapeutic aspects in management of patients with multiple sclerosis. *Diseases of the Nervous System*, **21**, 24–6.

Browning WN. (1990) Exacerbation of symptoms of multiple sclerosis in a patient taking fluoxetine. *American Journal of Psychiatry*, **147**, 1089.

Charcot JM. (1877) *Lectures on the Diseases of the Nervous System delivered at La Salpetriere*. pp. 194–5. New Sydenham Society: London.

Crawford JD, McIvor, GP. (1985) Group psychotherapy: benefits in multiple sclerosis. *Archives of Physical Medical Rehabilitation*, **66**, 810–13.

Dalos NP, Rabins PV, Brooks BR, O'Donnell P. (1983) Disease activity and emotional state in multiple sclerosis. *Annals of Neurology*, **13**, 573–7.

Day M, Day E, Herrmann R. (1953) Group therapy of patients with multiple sclerosis. *Archives of Neurology and Psychiatry*, **69**, 193–6.

Endicott J, Spitzer R. (1978) A diagnostic interview: the schedule for affective disorders and schizophrenia (SADS). *Archives of General Psychiatry*, **35**, 837–44.

Endicott J, Spitzer R. (1979) Use of the research diagnostic criteria and the schedule for affective disorders and schizophrenia to study affective disorders. *American Journal of Psychiatry*, **136**, 52–6.

Fassbender K, Schmidt R, Mößner R et al. (1998) Mood disorders and dysfunction of the hypothalamic–pituitary–adrenal axis in multiple sclerosis. *Archives of Neurology*, **55**, 66–72.

Feighner JP, Robins E, Guze SB, Woodruff RA, Winokur G, Munoz R. (1972) Diagnostic criteria for use in psychiatric research. *Archives of General Psychiatry*, **26**, 57–63.

Feinstein A. (1995) Multiple sclerosis and depression: an etiological conundrum. Canadian *Journal of Psychiatry*, **40**, 573–6.

Feinstein A. (1997) Multiple sclerosis, depression and suicide. *British Medical Journal*, **315**, 691–2.

Feinstein A, Youl B, Ron MA. (1992a) Acute optic neuritis: a cognitive and magnetic resonance imaging study. *Brain*, **115**, 1403–15.

Feinstein A, Kartsounis L, Miller B, Youl B, Ron MA. (1992b) Clinically isolated lesions of the type seen in multiple sclerosis: a cognitive, psychiatric and MRI follow-up study. *Journal of Neurology, Neurosurgery and Psychiatry*, **55**, 869–76.

Feinstein A, Ron MA, Thompson A. (1993) A serial study of psychometric and magnetic resonance imaging changes in multiple sclerosis. *Brain*, **116**, 569–602.

Flax JW, Gray J, Herbert J. (1991) Effects of fluoxetine on patients with multiple sclerosis. *American Journal of Psychiatry*, **148**, 1603.

Foley FW, Bedell JR, LaRocca NG, Scheinberg LC, Reznikoff M. (1987) Efficacy of Stress-Inoculation Training in coping with multiple sclerosis. *Journal of Consulting and Clinical Psychology*, **55**, 919–22.

Foley FW, Traugott U, LaRocca NG et al. (1992) A prospective study of depression and immune dysregulation in multiple sclerosis. *Archives of Neurology*, **49**, 238–44.

Gallineck A, Kalinowsky LB. (1958) Psychiatric aspects of multiple sclerosis. *Diseases of the Nervous System*, **19**, 77–80.

Gershon ES, Hamovit J, Guroff JJ et al. (1982) A family study of schizoaffective, bipolar 1, bipolar 11, unipolar, and normal control probands. *Archives of General Psychiatry*, **39**, 1157–67.

Goldberg DP, Blackwell BB. (1970) Psychiatric illness in general practice. A detailed study using a new method of case identification. *British Medical Journal*, **ii**, 439–43.

Honer WG, Hurwitz T, Li DKB, Palmer M, Paty DW. (1987) Temporal lobe involvement in multiple sclerosis patients with psychiatric disorders. *Archives of Neurology*, **44**, 187–90.

Huber SJ, Paulsen GW, Shuttleworth EC et al. (1987) Magnetic resonance imaging correlates of dementia in multiple sclerosis. *Archives of Neurology*, **44**, 732–6.

Joffe RT, Lippert GP, Gray TA, Sawa G, Horvath Z. (1987a) Mood disorder and multiple sclerosis. *Archives of Neurology*, **44**, 376–8.

Joffe RT, Lippert GP, Gray TA, Sawa G, Horvath Z. (1987b) Personal and family history of affective disorder, *Journal of Affective Disorders*, **12**, 63–5.

Johansson B, Roos B-E. (1974) 5–Hydroxyindoleacetic acid and homovanillic acid in cerebrospinal fluid of patients with neurological disease. *European Neurology*, **11**, 37–45.

Kahana E, Leibowitz U, Alter M. (1971) Cerebral multiple sclerosis. *Neurology*, **21**, 1179–85.

Kessler RC, McGonagle KA, Shanyang Z et al. (1994) Lifetime and 12 month prevalence of DSM-111–R psychiatric disorders in the United States. Results from the National Co-morbidity Survey. *Archives of General Psychiatry*, **51**, 8–19.

Krupp LB, Alvarez LA, LaRocca NG, Scheinberg LC. (1988) Fatigue in multiple sclerosis. *Archives of Neurology*, **45**, 435–7.

Krystal AD, Coffey CE. (1997) Neuropsychiatric considerations in the use of electroconvulsive therapy. *Journal of Neuropsychiatry and Clinical Neurosciences*, **9**, 283–92.

Kurtzke JF. (1983) Rating neurologic impairment in multiple sclerosis: an expanded disability scale. *Neurology*, **33**, 1444–52.

Larcombe NA, Wilson PH. (1984) An evaluation of cognitive-behaviour therapy for depression in patients with multiple sclerosis. *British Journal of Psychiatry*, **145**, 366–71.

Linde K, Ramirez G, Mulrow CD, Pauls A, Weidenhammer W, Melchart D. (1996) St. John's wort for depression – an overview and meta-analysis of randomised clinical trials. *British Medical Journal*, **313**, 253–8.

Logsdail SJ, Callanan MM, Ron MA. (1988) Psychiatric morbidity in patients with clinically isolated lesions of the type seen in multiple sclerosis. *Psychological Medicine*, **18**, 355–64.

Lyon-Caen O, Jouvent R, Hauser S et al. (1986) Cognitive function in recent onset demyelinating disease. *Archives of Neurology*, **43**, 1138–41.

Mathews WB. (1979) Multiple sclerosis presenting with acute remitting psychiatric symptoms. *Journal of Neurology, Neurosurgery and Psychiatry*, **42**, 859–63.

Mattingley G, Baker K, Zorumski CF, Figiel GS. (1992) Multiple sclerosis and ECT: possible value of gadolinium enhanced magnetic resonance scans for identifying high risk patients. *The Journal of Neuropsychiatry and Clinical Neurosciences*, **4**,

145–51.

Mayberg HS, Starkstein SE, Peyser CE et al. (1992) Paralimbic frontal lobe hypometabolism in depression associated with Huntington's Disease. *Neurology*, **42**, 1791–7.

Mayberg HS, Starkstein SE, Sadzot B et al. (1990) Selective hypometabolism in the inferior frontal lobe in depressed patients with Parkinson's disease. *Annals of Neurology*, **28**, 57–64.

McIvor GP, Riklan M, Reznikoff M. (1984) Depression in multiple sclerosis as a function of length and severity of illness, age, remissions and perceived social support. *Journal of Clinical Psychology*, **40**, 1028–33.

Michelson D, Stone L, Galliven E et al. (1994) Multiple sclerosis is associated with alterations in hypothalamic–pituitary–adrenal axis function. *Journal of Clinical Endocrinology and Metabolism*, **79**, 848–53.

Minden SL. (1992) Psychotherapy for people with multiple sclerosis. *Journal of Neuropsychiatry*, **4**, 198–213.

Minden SL, Schiffer RB. (1990) Affective disorders in multiple sclerosis. Review and recommendations for clinical research. *Archives of Neurology*, **47**, 98–104.

Minden SL, Orav J, Reich P. (1987) Depression in multiple sclerosis. *General Hospital Psychiatry*, **9**, 426–34.

Mohr DC, Goodkin DE, Likosky W, Gatto N, Baumann KA, Rudick RA. (1997) Treatment of depression improves adherance to interferon Beta-1b therapy for multiple sclerosis. *Archives of Neurology*, **54**, 531–3.

Neilly LK, Goodkin DS, Goodkin DE, Mohr DC, Hauser SL. (1996) Side effect profile of interferon beta-1B (Betaseron). *Neuroloy*, **46**, 552–4,

Nyenhuis DL, Rao SM, Zajecka JM, Luchetta T, Bernardin L, Garron DC. (1995) Mood disturbance versus other symptoms of depression in multiple sclerosis. *Journal of the International Neuropsychological Society*, **1**, 291–6.

Pavlou M, Johnson P, Davis FA., Lefebre K. (1979) Program of psychologic service delivery in multiple sclerosis centre. *Professional Psychologist*, **10**, 503–10.

Paykel ES, Myers JK, Lindethal JJ, Tanner J. (1974) Suicidal feelings in the general population: a prevalence study. *British Journal of Psychiatry*, **124**, 460–9.

Pujol J, Bello J, Deus J, Marti-Vilalta JL, Capdevila A. (1997) Lesions in the left arcuate fasciculus region and depressive symptoms in multiple sclerosis. *Neurology*, **49**, 1105–10.

Rabins PV, Brooks BR, O'Donnell P et al. (1986) Structural brain correlates of emotional disorder in multiple sclerosis. *Brain*, **109**, 585–97.

Rao SM, Leo GJ, Haughton VM, St. Aubin-Faubert P, Bernardin L. (1989) Correlation of magnetic resonance imaging with neuropsychological testing in multiple sclerosis. *Neurology*, **39**, 161–6.

Reder AT, Lowy MT, Meltzer HY, Antel JP. (1987) Dexamethasone suppression test abnormalities in multiple sclerosis: relation to ACTH therapy. *Neurology*, **37**, 849–53.

Reischies FM, Baum K, Brau H, Hedde JP, Schwindt G. (1988) Cerebral magnetic resonance imaging findings in multiple sclerosis. Relation to disturbance of affect, drive and cognition. *Archives of Neurology*, **45**, 1114–16.

Robinson RG, Kubos KL, Starr LB, Rao K, Price TR. (1983) Mood disorders in stroke patients: relationship to lesion location. *Comprehensive Psychiatry*, **24**, 555–6.

Ron MA, Logsdail SJ. (1989) Psychiatric morbidity in multiple sclerosis: a clinical and MRI study. *Psychological Medicine*, **19**, 887–95.

Rush AJ, Beck A, Kovacs M, Hollon SD. (1977) Comparative efficacy of cognitive therapy and pharmacotherapy in the treatment of depressed out-patients. *Cognitive therapy and Research*, **1**, 17–37.

Sadovnik AD, Eisen RN, Ebers GC, Paty DW. (1991) Cause of death in patients attending multiple sclerosis clinics. *Neurology*, **41**, 1193–6.

Sadovnik AD, Remick RA, Allen J et al. (1996) Depression and multiple sclerosis. *Neurology*, **46**, 628–32.

Sandyk R, Awerbuch G. (1993) Nocturnal melatonin secretion in suicidal patients with multiple sclerosis. *International Journal of Neuroscience*, **71**, 173–82.

Schiffer RB. (1987) The spectrum of depression in multiple sclerosis. An approach for clinical management. *Archives of Neurology*, **44**, 596–9.

Schiffer RB, Babigian HM. (1984) Behavioural disturbance in multiple sclerosis, temporal lobe epilepsy and amyotrophic lateral sclerosis; an epidemiologic study. *Archives of Neurology*, **41**, 1067–9.

Schiffer RB, Wineman NM. (1990) Antidepressant pharmacotherapy of depression associated with multiple sclerosis. *American Journal of Psychiatry*, **147**, 1493–7.

Schiffer RB, Caine ED, Bamford KA, Levy S. (1983) Depressive episodes in patients with multiple sclerosis. *American Journal of Psychiatry*, **140**, 1498–500.

Schiffer RB, Weitkamp LR, Wineman NM, Guttormsen S. (1988) Multiple sclerosis and affective disorder: family history, sex and HLA-DR antigens. *Archives of Neurology*, **45**, 1345–8.

Schubert DSP, Foliart RH. (1993) Increases depression in multiple sclerosis. A meta-analysis. *Psychosomatics*, **34**, 124–30.

Scott TF, Allen D, Price TRP, McConnell H, Lang D. (1996) Characterization of major depression symptoms in multiple sclerosis. *The Journal of Neuropsychiatry and Clinical Neurosciences*, **8**, 318–23.

Scott TF, Nussbaum P, McConnell H, Brill P. (1995) Measurement of treatment response to sertraline in depressed multiple sclerosis patients using the Carroll scale. *Neurological Research*, **17**, 421–2.

Shafey H. (1992) The effect of fluoxetine in depression associated with multiple sclerosis. *Canadian Journal of Psychiatry*, **37**, 147–8.

Shaw DM, Camps FE, Eccleston EG (1967) 5–hydroxytryptamine in the hindbrain of depressive suicides. *British Journal of Psychiatry*, **113**, 1407–11.

Skegg K, Corwin PA, Skegg DCG. (1988) How often is multiple sclerosis mistaken for a psychiatric disorder ? *Psychological Medicine*, **18**, 733–6.

Spielberg N. (1980) Support group improves quality of life. *Rehabilitation Nurses Journal*, **5**, 9–11.

Starkstein SE, Robinson RG. (1989) Affective disorders and cerebral vascular disease. *British Journal of Psychiatry*, **154**, 170–82.

Stenager E, Jensen K. (1988) Multiple sclerosis: correlation of psychiatric admissions to onset of initial symptoms. *Acta Neurologica Scandinavica*, **77**, 414–17.

Stenager EN, Stenager E. (1992) Suicide and patients with neurologic diseases. Methodologic problems. *Archives of Neurology*, **49**, 1296–303.

Stenager EN, Stenager E, Koch-Henrikson N, Brønnum-Hansen H, Hyllested K, Jensen K et al. (1992) Suicide and multiple sclerosis: an epidemiological investigation. *Journal of Neurology, Neurosurgery and Psychiatry*, **55**, 542–5.

Surridge D. (1969) An investigation into some aspects of multiple sclerosis. *British Journal of Psychiatry*, **115**, 749–64.

Thompson AJ, Miller D, Youl B et al. (1992) Serial gadolinium-enhanced MRI in relapsing/remitting multiple sclerosis of varying disease duration. *Neurology*, **42**, 60–3.

Wei T, Lightman SL. (1997) The neuroendocrine axis in patients with multiple sclerosis. *Brain*, **120**, 1067–76.

Whitlock FA, Siskind MM. (1980) Depression as a major symptom of multiple sclerosis. *Journal of Neurology, Neurosurgery and Psychiatry*, **43**, 861–5.

Young AC, Saunders J, Ponsford JR. (1976) Mental change as an early feature of multiple sclerosis. *Journal of Neurology, Neurosurgery and Psychiatry*, **39**, 1008–13.

3

Multiple sclerosis and bipolar affective disorder

Occasionally, it has been my experience to encounter a MS patient with mania, who apart from the abnormal mental state examination is neurologically quite well. Furthermore, I have treated patients with manic episodes heralding the onset of MS and have also come across bipolar patients who subsequently went on to develop MS often years later. I am struck by how much more common manic-psychosis is compared to a schizophrenia-type psychosis amongst MS patients, an observation supported by empirical research. Managing the floridly manic MS patient can present a considerable challenge given the potential that neuroleptic and mood stabilising medications have for further compromising neurological function. Early detection of the patient going 'high' makes management very much easier, but as a first step to early detection, increased awareness amongst clinicians of the increased rate of co-morbidity is needed. Criteria for diagnosing mania are well spelled out and as with clinically significant depression, diagnosis and treatment, particularly of the patients with mildly elevated mood does not have to await the arrival of a neuropsychiatrist.

Conceptual and semantic issues

Mania may occur as part of many physical conditions or as a reaction to drug therapy. When this occurs, the mania has been termed 'secondary', differentiating it from the more usual occurrence as a primary psychiatric syndrome. The correct DSM-1V (APA, 1994) terminology for the syndrome is a 'Mood disorder due to a general medical condition' (MDGMC)(Table 3.1), with the type of mood change specified as 'with manic features' (Table 3.2) or 'with hypomanic features' (Table 3.3). If the symptoms of mania are present together with depression and neither predominates, the type of mood change is specified as 'mixed'. The DSM-1V nomenclature has done away with the primary–secondary dichotomy, although the fundamental idea of the mood disorder arising as a result of the medical condition remains unchanged.

This terminology may be somewhat misleading. MS patients presenting with mania or hypomania are, more often than not, given the diagnosis of Bipolar Affective Disorder, Type 1 denoting mania and Type 11 hypomania. This has formerly been called Manic-Depressive Disorder in the earlier

Table 3.1. Diagnostic criteria for mood disorder (mania) due to a general medical condition

A.	A prominent and persistent disturbance in mood predominates in the clinical picture and is characterized by: an elevated, expansive or irritable mood
B.	There is evidence from the history, physical examination, or laboratory findings that the disturbance is the direct physiological consequence of the medical condition.
C.	The disturbance is not better accounted for by another mental disorder (e.g. a bipolar disorder that predates the medical condition by many years).
D.	The disturbance does not occur exclusively during the course of a delirium.
E.	The symptoms cause clinically significant distress or impairment in social, occupational, or other important areas of functioning. The *types* are then specified as either manic or mixed. The general medical condition should be mentioned on Axis 1 and should also be coded on Axis 3.

Reprinted with permission. © 1994 American Psychiatric Association.
The DSM-1V makes the point that, although the clinical presentation of the mood disorder may resemble a manic or hypomanic episode, the full criteria for one of these episodes need not be met (see Tables 3.2 and 3.3 for the full criteria for a manic or hypomanic episode).

Table 3.2. Criteria for a manic episode

A.	A distinct period of abnormally and persistently elevated, expansive or irritable mood lasting at least 1 week (or any duration if hospitalization is necessary).
B.	During the period of mood disturbance, three or more of the following symptoms have persisted (four if the mood is only irritable) and have been present to a significant degree: (i) inflated self-esteem or grandiosity (ii) decreased need for sleep (e.g. feels rested after only 3 hours of sleep) (iii) more talkative than usual or pressure to keep talking (iv) flight of ideas or subjective experience that thoughts are racing (v) distractibility (i.e. attention too easily drawn to unimportant or irrelevant external stimuli) (vi) increase in goal-directed activity (either socially, at work or school, or sexually) or psychomotor agitation (vii) excessive involvement in pleasurable activities that have a high potential for painful consequences (e.g. engaging in unrestrained buying sprees, sexual indiscretions, or foolish business investments)
C.	The mood disturbance is sufficiently severe to cause marked impairment in occupational functioning or in usual social activities or relationships with others, or to necessitate hospitalization to prevent harm to self or others, or there are psychotic features.

Reprinted with permission. © 1994 American Psychiatric Association.

Table 3.3. Criteria for a hypomanic episode

A.	A distinct period of persistently elevated, expansive or irritable mood lasting throughout at least 4 days, that is clearly different from the usual non-depressed mood.
B.	As in the criteria for manic episode.
C.	The episode is associated with an unequivocal change in functioning that is uncharacteristic of the person when not symptomatic.
D.	The disturbance in mood and the change in functioning are observable by others.
E.	The episode is not severe enough to cause marked impairment in social or occupational functioning, or to necessitate hospitalisation and there are no psychotic features.

Reprinted with permission. © 1994 American Psychiatric Association.

World Health Organization classifications of mental illness. Confusion is understandable as the signs and symptoms of Bipolar Affective Disorder are indistinguishable from MDGMC; manic subtype. Thus, the situation with respect to terminology bears many similarities to that found in depression (see Chapter 2) and psychosis (see Chapter 5). For the purposes of this chapter, mania in the context of MS will be referred to as Bipolar Affective Disorder, even though this is not strictly correct by the criteria of the DSM-1V. The decision is nevertheless a practical one, because the literature makes reference overwhelmingly to Bipolar Affective Disorder and not MDGMC. The DSM-1V is, however, only 5 years old, and future research may see a change in this regard.

This chapter will review briefly the literature pertaining to Bipolar Affective Disorder and medical conditions in general, before the focus shifts specifically to MS. The epidemiology, etiology and treatment of mania in the context of MS will be discussed and a section is devoted to differential diagnosis, in particular the mental state change of euphoria.

Literature review of mania and medical illness

In a wide-ranging review of the disorder, Krauthammer and Klerman (1978) found cases of mania occurring in association with infection, neoplasm, epilepsy and metabolic disturbances. Drugs implicated included corticosteroids, isoniazid, procarbazine, levodopa and bromide. No cases of multiple sclerosis were reported. Using criteria more restrictive than current DSM-1V guidelines for a mood disorder due to a general medical condition (i.e. manic symptoms had to be present for longer than a week) the authors identified certain characteristics of mania that suggested a link to the associated medical disorder. These included a later age of onset of mania, which in their review was on average 41 years (as opposed to 25 years in 'primary' bipolar illness) and the relative absence of a family history of affective illness. Written during an era when psychiatric disorders were divided into either organic or functional, Krauthammer and Klerman (1978) concluded that secondary mania was organic in origin.

Their observations were replicated in a study comprising 39 manic patients with and without an antecedent medical illness (Cook et al., 1987). Additional differences in the medically ill sample included a predominantly irritable mood, more assaultative behaviour, less Schneiderian first rank symptoms and more personality change. Once again, the sample did not contain patients with MS.

MS and bipolar affective disorder

Prevalence of co-morbidity

Over the years there have been case reports of mania associated with MS (Peselow et al., 1981; Garfield, 1985; Kwentus et al., 1986). In addition, two patients with rapid cycling bipolar disorder and multiple sclerosis have been reported (Kellner et al., 1984). In the patient described by Kwentus et al. (1986), mania was the only clinical manifestation of disease activity and occurred together with abnormal changes in the CSF cell count. While clinically informative, these case reports have not been able to address the issue of whether the co-occurrence of MS and mania exceeds chance expectation.

One study that purported to show this was Hutchinson et al. (1993), who described a series of seven patients whose bipolar disorder, either presenting as recurrent manic episodes or mania alternating with depression, appeared many years before the onset of their neurological symptoms. The patients were collected over a 10–year period and were part of a database of 550 MS patients, which yielded a prevalence rate of antecedent bipolar disorder in MS of 1.2%. Five of the ten patients had had MRI brain scans during their initial psychiatric assessment and they all revealed white matter changes compatible with a diagnosis of MS, although two of the cases also had marked cerebral atrophy. Based on these findings, the authors concluded that mania may, in some patients, be a presenting symptoms of MS. This does not, however, fit with the DSM-1V concept of a temporal association between the medical and psychiatric conditions. In addition, it is unclear to what extent the 550 patients in the database were representative of MS patients in general and, as such, ascertainment bias cannot be ruled out.

Firmer evidence of an increased association between the two disorders comes from a study in Monroe County, New York. Schiffer et al. (1986) attempted to trace all patients in the county (population 702 238) who had both MS and Bipolar Affective Disorder. Patients were excluded if their manic episode occurred in the context of corticosteroid treatment. Assuming lifetime risks of 0.77% and 100/100 000 for Bipolar Disorder and MS, respectively, the expected rate of comorbidity was estimated to be 5.4. However, twice the number of patients were found to have both conditions. In all cases demyelination preceded the first affective symptom by at least 1 year. While the absence of a more immediate temporal association between the disorders is once again problematic, the representative nature of the sample studied provides more robust evidence of a link. Indeed, Schiffer et al. (1986) acknowledge that their figure may, in fact, be an underestimate of the true co-morbidity because cases of either disorder may not have appeared on the computerized records kept in the county, while in addition, MS may have shortened the lifespan of individuals, thereby decreasing the observed prevalence rate of patients with both conditions.

Joffe et al. (1987a) supported these conclusions. One hundred consecutive MS clinic attenders were interviewed with the Schedule for Affective Disorders and Schizophrenia lifetime version that enabled diagnoses compatible with DSM-111 criteria to be made. Patients had to have a history of depression and hypomania and sought psychiatric help before a diagnosis of bipolar disorder was given. Despite these strict selection criteria, 13% of patients were found to have a lifetime prevalence of bipolar disorder, well in excess of the 1% rate in the general population. Given the small sample size and ascertainment bias (the clinic was part of a tertiary referral process) Joffe et al.'s figure is likely to be an overestimate, but even making allowances for these limitations, the result still points to an increased prevalence of mania associated with MS.

Indirect evidence confirming an increased association comes from a study of 2720 psychiatric inpatients screened for MS. Although only ten patients with MS were detected, they were more likely to present with manic or hypomanic symptoms than the remainder of the inpatient sample (Pine et al., 1995). In common with Hutchinson et al.'s (1993) series, almost two-thirds of patients had had psychiatric admissions before going on to receive a diagnosis of MS.

Etiology of bipolar disorder in MS

Research in this area is limited, but has focused on three aspects, a genetic vulnerability, adverse reactions to steroids, and regional brain changes demonstrated by MRI.

Genetics

Schiffer et al. (1986) in their Monroe County study found that five of their ten bipolar patients had first- or second-degree relatives with a clinically significant affective disorder, while one patient had a family history of schizophrenia. The authors did not comment on what, at first sight, seems to be an increased genetic loading for mental illness. No distinction was made between a family history of unipolar or bipolar depression, and the comparable figures for the MS patients without affective disorders were not given. However, in another study that specifically addressed the question of genetic vulnerability to mood change in MS, Schiffer et al. (1988) investigated 56 patients with MS, divided into four groups, namely bipolar (n=15), unipolar (n=16), no affective disorder (n=13) and probably no affective disorder (n=12). Sufficient data were available in 44 of these patients allowing conclusions to be drawn about a family history of mental illness. Two-thirds of the bipolar MS patients had a family history of affective disorder as opposed to one of the 16 unipolar MS patients and two of the 13 MS patients without affective disorders, the differences between the bipolar and unipolar patients proving statistically significant. In addition, five of the 44 patients had a family history of MS. Of these, four were bipolar and one unipolar and while these numbers were small, they reinforced the conclusion that a genetic link was present between MS and affective disorder, predominantly of a bipolar subtype.

Schiffer and colleagues extended their analysis to look at the effects of gender on mood and found that three of the 15 bipolar probands and one of the 16 unipolar probands were male. Controlling for a known female bias in MS (ratio of 1.5–2 females to 1 male) females with MS were still statistically more likely to have an affective disorder than males. Among the 34 affectively ill relatives of the probands, the proportion of males and females affected was equal, but when the disorders were split into unipolar or bipolar, female and male predilections for bipolar and unipolar disorders, respectively, were noted. An attempt to further validate these findings by looking for associations with various HLA antigen subtypes was inconclusive, the small sample size preventing meaningful statistical analysis. Although this line of research appeared to offer potentially useful clues as to the familial transmission of affective disorder in MS, in particular bipolar disorder, no further attempts have been made to replicate or extend the findings.

Contradictory results were, however, reported by another study looking at familial risk. Joffe et al. (1987b) used the family history method to assess the prevalence of affective disorders in the probands of affected MS patients. No excess of affective disorders was found in the relatives, leading the authors to suggest mood change in MS was an intrinsic part of the neurological disorder.

Steroid induced mania

The mood altering properties of steroids and ACTH are well known, and mild to moderate degrees of mania may occur in up to a third of patients (Ling et al., 1981). Minden et al. (1988), in a retrospective study, investigated steroid-induced mania in a sample of 50 patients with MS. Although they could not determine dosage, duration of treatment, or response to treatment from the case notes, the authors were able to interview informants to ascertain: (a) whether the medication was in fact taken, (b) the intervals between starting the medication and the development of psychiatric symptoms, and (c) the duration between stopping the treatment and the cessation of mania. Psychiatric symptomatology and diagnoses were made using the Schedule for Affective Disorders and Schizophrenia lifetime version which generated Research Diagnostic Criteria diagnoses. Nine patients developed mania or hypomania (at least 1 week of elevated or irritable mood and increased activity of various forms) during the course of their treatment. There was a close temporal relationship between symptom onset/resolution and treatment starting and ending. In one patient the elevated mood persisted and worsened in time, ending in a full-blown manic state with psychotic features that gradually subsided into a depressive disorder on discontinuation of the ACTH.

A search for clinical predictors of mania was limited to the ACTH group as they were more likely to become manic than the prednisone-treated patients. The most striking finding was that a history of major depression either before or after the diagnosis of MS, or a family history of unipolar depression, or alcoholism or both were risk factors for patients becoming manic. There were no differences between the manic and non-manic patients on any demographic or disease-related variables. In addition, manic symptoms did not occur with every drug exposure. Although the study was not without methodological problems, in particular the retrospective nature of the data collected, the evidence suggested that risk factors for mania include ACTH as opposed to prednisone and a premorbid and/or genetic diathesis for psychopathology, particularly depression or alcoholism.

The prophylactic nature of lithium therapy in corticotrophin-induced mania (Falk et al., 1979) means that physicians should not necessarily discontinue treatment if patients become high. Rather, the careful monitoring of the mental state on a reduced dose of ACTH, together with the addition of lithium, may allow treatment to continue.

Cerebral correlates of mania

Before discussing the MRI brain changes reported in manic MS patients, a summary of the MRI findings in bipolar patients without a neurological illness is required. The most replicated findings are those of white matter and periventricular hyperintensities, while the evidence linking bipolar disorders to more regional brain pathology, in particular, abnormalities in the limbic structures of the temporal lobes, is more equivocal. Similarly, the support for any definite cerebral laterality effect is inconclusive. The literature has been reviewed by Soares and Mann (1997), who also noted some evidence of a larger third ventricle and perhaps a smaller temporal lobe volume in bipolar patients.

The MRI finding of periventricular white matter lesions has certain similarities with MS, and the possibility of the two disorders having a shared etiology (Young et al., 1997), or that bipolar disorder arises from anomalous myelination (Dupont et al., 1995), has been suggested. Such views, however, lack substance. While there are some imaging similarities in a subset of patients, there are also many more substantial differences. MRI brain changes are virtually ubiquitous in MS, which is not the case in bipolar disorders. In addition, the pathology of the white matter lesions in bipolar patients has not been established. At present, a vascular etiology is favoured (Soares and Mann, 1997). MRI may therefore have good sensitivity in detecting white matter changes, but it lacks the specificity to determine etiology.

No neuroimaging study has addressed the specific question of cerebral changes in manic MS patients. In a MRI study of psychosis in MS, Feinstein et al. (1992) noted the presence of increased plaque in the regions surrounding the temporal horns of psychotic as opposed to non-psychotic MS patients. The psychotic sample was equally divided between affective and schizophrenia-like presentations and there were no MRI differences between them. As there is no evidence that the disease process in MS selectively targets these areas, the authors suggested the lesion burden or white matter loss in the temporal lobes may have to exceed a putative critical threshold in patients with a prior diathesis for mood disorders, before clinical symptoms are triggered.

There is little in the literature to substantiate or refute this view. Of the five manic patients who underwent MRI of the brain in Hutchinson et al.'s (1993) series, only one had lesions in the temporal lobes. Reischies et al. (1988) looked at the relationship between MRI brain changes and individual psychiatric symptoms and reported that periventricular and frontal white matter lesions were closely associated with poor judgement and euphoria. However, their study had a number of shortcomings, such as a failure to use valid and reliable methods of rating psychiatric symptoms, and consequently the absence of psychiatric diagnoses. Thus, whether the observed changes in mood and judgement were part of a manic illness could not be ascertained. Finally, Casanova et al. (1996) confirmed at postmortem the presence of marked, diffuse periventricular demyelination in a 81–year-old female with late onset mania, whose neurological examination had been normal over a 31–year period. Although the case report highlights the possibility of mania alone being a symptom of MS, a predominantly periventricular lesion distribution in an elderly patient is too non-specific to be regarded as a firm cerebral correlate of mania.

Differential diagnosis

Although the diagnosis of a hypomanic or manic episode is often straightforward, two other clinical disorders may prove potentially misleading. Hypomania must be differentiated from euphoria and mania with psychotic features should be distinguished from a non-affective psychosis.

Euphoria

For many years, euphoria was considered virtually pathognomonic of the abnormal mental state in MS. In an influential early paper, Cottrell and Wilson (1926) reported it in over two-thirds of their sample and defined four states, namely 'mental wellbeing' or 'euphoria sclerotica' characterized by a persistently cheerful mood; 'physical wellbeing' or eutonia sclerotica distinguished by unconcern over physical disability; 'pes sclerotica', an incongruous optimism for the future; and emotional lability. Although the validity of such an approach has never been adequately proven, the above criteria, with the exception of emotional lability, are still considered pathognomonic of the condition. Thus, as currently defined, euphoria bears some similarity to hypomania with regard to elevated affect, but lacks the associated motor overactivity and increased energy manifesting as a flurry of new ideas and activities. Euphoria is fixed rather than fluctuating, may best be considered akin to a personality change, and this clinical picture is, for the most part, readily discernable from hypomania (Surridge, 1970).

Few studies since Cottrell and Wilson (1926) have reported such high rates. Surridge (1969), comparing his case register of MS patients to a control group with muscular dystrophy (MD) found euphoria in 26% of the MS as opposed to none of the MD group. Poser (1980) reported a 24% rate while Rabins et al. (1986), using Cottrell and Wilson's (1926) definition noted a 48% point prevalence. A reason for the decline in frequency has been the recognition that many patients with emotional lability appear superficially euphoric, but in reality have subjective evidence of depressed mood. In addition, those subjects with emotional incontinence (also termed pathological laughing and crying) that were included in Cottrell and Wilson's rubric of emotional wellbeing, are now considered a distinct entity (see Chapter 4). Summarizing the various studies to date, a median rate of 25% probably accurately reflects the true prevalence of euphoria (Rabins, 1990).

Euphoria is considered a manifestation of advanced MS, commensurate with extensive cerebral damage. Studies demonstrating an association with greater physical disability and cognitive impairment (Surridge, 1969; Rabins et al., 1986), progressive disease course and enlarged ventricles on CT (Rabins et al., 1986), frontal lesions (Reischies et al., 1988) and more widespread lesions (Ron and Logsdail, 1989) on MRI, have all been reported.

Non-affective psychosis

Differentiating a psychotic manic patient from a patient with a non-affective psychosis may also present a clinical challenge, as the latter may display considerable agitation and emotional arousal, leading to an erroneous impression of mania. It is, however, the prominence and persistence of mood change that suggests an affective diagnosis.

The importance of establishing the correct diagnosis is self-evident, determining both the treatment and prognosis.

Treatment

A 34-year-old married female on long-term disability payments because of a 5-year history of MS (EDSS of 5.5) was brought to the emergency room by her husband in the small hours of the morning. The police were in attendance as their help had been required to bring the patient into hospital. The husband reported his wife had not slept for 4 nights, had recently spent a large sum of money using her credit card to shop by telephone and had started assaulting him with her walking stick. The patient appeared irritable and was hostile to questioning. She demanded an immediate release so that she could return home and pursue plans that were to make her a lot of money. When pressed to divulge these plans, she spoke of developing a game called 'FRAGILE', whereby the players had to make up new words using the letters contained in the word 'fragile'. She had been determined to teach the game to her 2-year-old daughter and frustrated by the child's inability to learn the procedure had beaten her.

A diagnosis of bipolar affective disorder: manic episode was made, the patient admitted to hospital and detained under a provision of the Mental Health Act. She refused all medication and had to be declared incapable of consenting to treatment. Her behaviour on the ward was dismissive and angry and her cane was confiscated because of assaults on the nursing staff. Without the cane, her ataxia worsened, but such was her degree of motor overactivity and manically driven behaviour, she refused a wheelchair or any form of assistance and had a number of falls. Sedation was needed and had to be given by the intramuscular route. Lorazepam 1–2 mg were injected four times per day as required. This sedated the patient, but produced further unsteadiness, leaving her at added risk of falling. A nursing assistant was therefore assigned to remain constantly with her. While the Lorazepam was effective in slowing the patient down, it did not produce a lessening in her grandiose delusional beliefs. A neuroleptic drug, haloperidol was therefore also given in a dose of 0.5 mg b.i.d. After 24 hours the dose was raised to 1 mg b.i.d. and after a further 4 days, the patient's irritability and grandiosity gradually began improving.

At this point she agreed to take medication orally. Lithium carbonate 300 mg t.i.d. was introduced, but the patient was unable to tolerate the drug because it exacerbated her urinary incontinence, thereby adding to her agitation. Sodium valproate was substituted and 250 mg given b.i.d. with food. At this point the haloporidol was gradually tapered off over the course of a week while the sodium valproate increased by increments of 250 mg until she was taking a dose of 500 mg b.i.d. Lorazepam was no longer required and 2 weeks after admission the patient's mood was judged to be euthymic and her thought content normal. She was on monotherapy and tolerating the sodium valproate well. She was discharged from hospital and given an outpatient follow-up. Three years later, she remains on sodium valproate, although the dose had to be increased to 500 mg t.i.d. to deal with a hypomanic episode.

This case presentation captures the many potential difficulties posed by treating the floridly manic MS patient and illustrates the range of drug treatments that may be required. Lesser degrees of mania, without psychosis, are easier to treat and frequently respond well to monotherapy in the form of a mood-stabilizing drug. Here, the clinician is faced with a number of choices, the most widely used being lithium carbonate, carbamazepine and sodium valproate. In more intractable cases, I have resorted to the use of the calcium channel blocker, verapamil, with variable success. More recently, the emergence of newer antiseizure drugs such as gabapentin and lamotrigine have also been reported to have mood-stabilizing properties, although their use in MS bipolar MS patients awaits clarification.

Of all the drugs available, the most data have accrued with respect to lithium. Although lithium is generally an effective treatment for mania in patients with neurological disease (Young et al., 1977), the data pertaining to its use in MS bipolar patients are limited, contradictory and anecdotal. There are no controlled treatment trials in manic MS patients. Kemp et al. (1977) and Solomon (1978) found the drug was effective while Kellner et al. (1984) and Kwentus et al. (1986) did not. As lithium is known to produce a diuresis, MS patients with bladder problems may have difficulty tolerating the drug. Furthermore, Solomon (1978) cautioned against mistaking the development of neurological impairment as a sign of lithium toxicity. Should the manic episode be suggestive of an exacerbation in a patient's MS, Peselow et al. (1981) endorse a combination of prednisone plus lithium. Should the mania be steroid induced, a dose reduction or the addition of lithium may prove helpful (Minden et al.,1988).

An alternative mood stabilizer is sodium valproate, which may be equally effective, but better tolerated (Stip and Daoust, 1995). As with lithium, there are no clinical trials providing empirical support for these anecdotal observations. Given that both MS and bipolar disorders may run relapsing–remitting courses, prophylaxis with mood-stabilizing drugs may be required for many years.

Should sedation be required for agitation, a benzodiazepine such as clonazepam is recommended. In the case of manic patients who become psychotic, neuroleptic treatment will often be required. There are no drug trials on which to base recommendations, but newer neuroleptics such as olanzapine and risperidone are effective and produce fewer side effects (in particular extrapyramidal symptoms that exacerbate pre-existing motor, balance and coordination difficulties) than the commonly used phenothiazines (e.g. chlorpromazine, perphenazine) and butyrophenones (e.g. haloperidol).

Finally, it is a rule of thumb that the clinician, when encountering a depressed MS patient, should always enquire about a past history of mania. Should there be one, the correct diagnosis is bipolar affective disorder and the treatment plan must be modified to include a mood-stabilizing drug, in addition to the required antidepressant.

Summary

- Bipolar affective disorder (manic episodes) in association with multiple sclerosis occur more frequently than chance expectation.
- The possibility of a shared genetic diathesis could explain the association, although preliminary results need replication.
- Both MS and bipolar disorder are associated with white matter changes on MRI, although the pathogenesis of these lesions is likely to be different.
- There is MRI evidence suggesting manic patients with psychosis have plaques that are distributed predominantly in bilateral temporal horn areas.
- MS patients who become hypomanic or manic on steroid therapy are more likely to have a family history of affective disorder and/or alcoholism or a premorbid psychiatric history of these disorders. This should not be a contraindication to treatment with steroids, although caution is advised.
- Lithium carbonate is an effective treatment for manic and hypomanic (including steroid induced) episodes. Sodium valproate is an effective alternative treatment for patients unable to tolerate lithium.
- Should mania be accompanied by psychosis, neuroleptic medication may be required. Benzodiazepines are useful as an adjunct for sedation.

References

American Psychiatric Association (1994) *Diagnostic and Statistical Manual of Mental Disorders*. Fourth Edition. American Psychiatric Associations: Washington, DC.

Casanova MF, Kruesi M, Mannheim G. (1996) Multiple sclerosis and bipolar disorder: a case report with autopsy findings. *Journal of Neuropsychiatry and Clinical Neurosciences*, **8**, 206–8.

Cook BL, Shukla S, Hoff AL, Aronson TA. (1987) Mania with associated organic factors. *Acta Psychiatrica Scandinavica*, **76**, 674–7.

Cottrell SS, Wilson SAK. (1926) The affective symptomatology of disseminated sclerosis. *Journal of Neurological Psychopathology*, **7**, 1–30.

Dupont RM, Jernigan TL, Heindel WN et al. (1995) Magnetic Resonance Imaging and mood disorders – localisation of white matter and other subcortical abnormalities. *Archives of General Psychiatry*, **52**, 747–55.

Falk WE, Mahnke MW, Poskanzer DC. (1979) Lithium prophylaxis of corticotrophin-induced psychosis. *Journal of the American Medical Association*, **241**, 1011–12.

Feinstein A, du Boulay G, Ron MA. (1992) Psychotic illness in multiple sclerosis. A clinical and magnetic resonance imaging study. *British Journal of Psychiatry*, **161**, 680–5.

Garfield DAS. (1985) Multiple sclerosis and affective disorder: 2 cases of mania with psychosis. *Psychotherapy and Psychosomatics*, **44**, 22–33.

Hutchinson M, Stack J, Buckley P. (1993) Bipolar affective disorder prior to the onset of multiple sclerosis. *Acta Neurologica Scandinavica*, **88**, 388–93.

Joffe RT, Lippert GP, Gray TA, Sawa G, Horvath Z. (1987a) Mood disorder and multiple sclerosis. *Archives of Neurology*, **44**, 376–8.

Joffe RT, Lippert GP, Gray TA, Sawa G, Horvath Z. (1987b) Personal and family history of affective illness in patients with multiple sclerosis. *Journal of Affective Disorders*, **12**, 63–5.

Kellner CH, Davenport Y, Post RM, Ross RJ. (1984) Rapid cycling bipolar disorder and multiple sclerosis. *American Journal of Psychiatry*, **141**, 112–13.

Kemp K, Lion JR, Magram G. (1977) Lithium in the case of of a manic patient with multiple sclerosis – a case report. *Diseases of the Nervous System*, **38**, 210–11.

Krauthammer C, Klerman GL. (1978) Secondary mania. Manic syndromes associated with antecedent physical illness and drugs. *Archives of General Psychiatry*, **35**, 1333–9.

Kwentus JA, Hart RP, Calabrese V, Hekmati A. (1986) Mania as a symptom of multiple sclerosis. *Psychosomatics*, **27**, 729–31.

Ling MHM, Perry PJ, Tsuang MT. (1981) Side effects of corticosteroid therapy. *Archives of General Psychiatry*, **38**, 471–7.

Minden SL, Schiffer RB. (1990) Affective disorders in multiple sclerosis. *Archives of Neurology*, **47**, 98–104.

Minden SL, Orav J, Schildkraut JJ. (1988) Hypomanic reactions to ACTH and prednisone treatment for multiple sclerosis. *Neurology*, **38**, 1631–4.

Peselow ED, Deutsch SI, Fieve RR, Kaufman M. (1981) Coexistent manic symptoms and multiple sclerosis. *Psychosomatics*, **22**, 824–5.

Pine DS, Douglas CJ, Charles E, Davies M, Kahn D. (1995) Patients with multiple sclerosis presenting to psychiatric hospitals. *Journal of Clinical Psychiatry*, **56**, 297–306.

Poser CM. (1980) Exacerbations, activity and progression in multiple sclerosis. *Archives of Neurology*, **37**, 471–4.

Rabins PV. (1990) Euphoria in multiple sclerosis. In *Neurobehavioural Aspects of*

Multiple Sclerosis, (ed. SM Rao), pp. 180–5. New York: Oxford University Press.

Rabins PV, Brooks BR, O'Donnell P et al. (1986) Structural brain correlates of emotional disorder in multiple sclerosis. *Brain*, **109**, 585–97.

Reischies FM, Baum K, Bräu H, Hedde JP, Schwindt G. (1988) Cerebral magnetic resonance imaging findings in multiple sclerosis. Relation to disturbance of affect, drive and cognition. *Archives of Neurology*, **45**, 1114–16.

Ron MA, Logsdail SJ. (1989) Psychiatric morbidity in multiple sclerosis: a clinical and MRI study. *Psychological Medicine*, **19**, 887–95.

Schiffer RB, Wineman M, Weitkamp LR. (1986) Association between bipolar affective disorder and multiple sclerosis. *American Journal of Psychiatry*, **143**, 94–5.

Schiffer RB, Weitkamp LR, Wineman M, Guttormsen S. (1988) Multiple sclerosis and affective disorder. Family history, sex and HLA-DR antigens. *Archives of Neurology*, **45**, 1345–8.

Soares JC, Mann JJ. (1997) The anatomy of mood disorders-Review of Structural Neuroimaging studies. *Biological Psychiatry*, **41**, 86–106.

Solomon JG. (1978) Multiple sclerosis masquerading as lithium toxicity. The *Journal of Nervous and Mental Disease*, **166**, 663–5.

Stip E, Daoust L. (1995) Valproate in the treatment of mood disorder due to multiple sclerosis. *Canadian Journal of Psychiatry*, **40**, 219–20.

Surridge D. (1969) An investigation into some psychiatric aspects of multiple sclerosis. *British Journal of Psychiatry*, **115**, 749–64.

Young LD, Taylor I, Holmstrom V. (1977) Lithium treatment of patients with affective illness associated with organic brain symptoms. *American Journal of Psychiatry*, **134**, 1405–7.

Young CR, Weiss EL, Bowers MB, Mazure CM. (1997) The differential diagnosis of multiple sclerosis and bipolar affective disorder. *Journal of Clinical Psychiatry*, **58**, 123.

4

Multiple sclerosis and pathological laughing and crying

Pathological Laughing and Crying (PLC) has been described with diverse neurological disorders, such as Alzheimer's disease (Starkstein et al., 1995), stroke (Morris et al., 1993), cerebral tumours (Monteil and Cohadon, 1996), amyotrophic lateral sclerosis (Gallagher, 1989) and multiple sclerosis (Minden and Schiffer, 1990). Most of the research on PLC in MS was completed prior to 1970, and the studies are beset by problems with methodology. Of the five pre-1970 papers, only Cottrell and Wilson's (1926) frequently cited article was devoted exclusively to the topic, the remainder discussing PLC in the context of other mental state abnormalities occurring in MS. Thus, inattention to detail, coupled with methodological shortcomings, has meant that the limited literature devoted to the syndrome has been inconsistent and, at times, misleading.

Review of earlier studies

Cottrell and Wilson (1926) studied 100 cases of MS seen in a tertiary referral centre. They developed a standardized interview of 44 questions probing patients mood, thoughts, somatic complaints and affect. The separation of mood and affect made the important distinction that what patients subjectively felt was not necessarily mirrored by what could be objectively noted. The study contained a wealth of descriptive data, such as demographic characteristics, the duration of neurological symptoms, and physical disability according to predominant system involvement (i.e. cerebellar, spinal, etc.). Abnormalities of affect were divided into three categories termed, 'euphoria sclerotica', 'eutonia sclerotica' and 'pes sclerotica', respectively. The first referred to a mood of serenity and cheerfulness, the second to a sense of somatic wellbeing despite physical disability, and the third to an incongruous and misplaced optimism of eventual full recovery from the MS.

The study's most notable finding was that 63% of patients had euphoria and 10% depression. A further 25% were noted to have increased variability in mood since the onset of MS. Thus, the overwhelming majority of patients had experienced a disordered mood since the onset of demyelination. With regard to a sense of physical wellbeing ('eutonia sclerotica'), this was endorsed by 84% of patients.

It was, however, Cottrell and Wilson's comments on affect that are germane to PLC. Of their sample 95% were deemed to have various degrees of pathological affect; 71% smiling and laughing constantly, 19% with mixed smiling and laughing plus crying, 2% displaying rapid shifts from laughing to crying and 3% crying constantly. These signs were noticeable for occurring 'in season and out of season, under slight provocation, at the bidding of minimal stimuli and make their appearance when there is certainly no obvious warrant for them'. A more conservative reading of the study suggests that, in only half the patients was the emotional display inappropriate, something the authors also acknowledge. No association was noted with the degree of physical disability, duration of illness, or grouping of neurological symptoms. Another important observation was the presence of outward displays of happiness unmatched by comparable, subjective feelings. The authors concluded that 'emotional facility and overaction form one of the cardinal features of the disease'.

The study was important for it was the first to investigate the problem of PLC in MS in considerable detail. However, there were a number of flaws that compromised the validity of the conclusions. Patients were seen at a tertiary referral centre and no details were given about how cases were selected. Thus, the sample was unlikely to reflect a representative group of patients with MS. Furthermore, the interview to ascertain whether emotional difficulties were present had not been validated and there was a failure to adequately define 'pathological laughing or crying'. While definitions were supplied for terms such as 'euphoria sclerotica' and 'eutonia sclerotica', these were not necessarily synonymous with PLC. This failure to define exactly what constituted the syndrome of PLC was to bedevil subsequent studies too. It is, however, important to view Cottrell and Wilson's findings in a historical context. Judged by the more rigorous standards applied to research methodology today, the weaknesses are apparent. But, the study served an important function by focusing attention on mentation in patients with MS, and highlighted the fact that disturbances in affect are common.

Langworthy et al. (1941) in a study of behavioural abnormalities seen in 199 patients with MS attending an outpatient clinic noted that, in the later stages of the disease, some patients presented with uncontrollable laughter and/or crying. They regarded the condition as part of pseudobulbar palsy and postulated a freeing of bulbar mechanisms from cortical control. Thirteen patients displayed the phenomenon, establishing a point prevalence of 6.5%, considerably lower than Cottrell and Wilson's figure. The majority of their patients displayed uncontrollable crying, with some patients alternating rapidly between the two states. The authors stressed that pathological laughing (PL) should be regarded as distinct from euphoria, but then equivocated and wondered whether the latter was not perhaps a mild variant of forced laughing. Nevertheless, the distinction between PL and euphoria accounts, at least in part, for the substantially different prevalence rates between this study and Cottrell and Wilson's earlier effort.

The definition of 'emotional dyscontrol' was subsequently loosened by Sugar and Nadell (1943). Their sample consisted of 28 inpatients, all with longstanding MS, of whom 43% displayed constant smiling and laughing, 25% had a mixed picture (smiling, laughing and crying), 4% changed rapidly between the two states and 7% cried constantly. Overall, 79% of their patients were deemed to have exaggerated emotional expression. The study suffered from the same methodological limitations as Cottrell and Wilson's, without the virtue of good sample size.

In a wide-ranging investigation of psychiatric aspects of MS, Pratt (1951) selected 100 outpatients with MS, excluding those with more advanced disease. Once again, the interview formulated by Cottrell and Wilson was used, but the study differed in using a control group of 100 patients, all but three having 'organic disease of the nervous system'. The disorders that constituted the control group were not revealed, but patients and controls were matched for age and gender. MS patients were found to laugh ($n=22$) and cry ($n=29$) more easily, giving a 51% prevalence rate for pathological affect. Although Pratt excluded very neurologically disabled cases, he concluded that impaired control over laughing and crying was more often associated with a more severe degree of physical disability and intellectual impairment.

Finally, Surridge (1969) compared psychiatric abnormalities in 108 MS patient and 39 patients with muscular dystrophy. The latter were chosen as a control group because of the debilitating nature of their disease, despite a sparing of cerebral involvement. By controlling for the effects of disability, attribution of psychopathology could be assigned either to cerebral or reactive causes. Although the principle was a sound one, any advantage was offset by applying arbitrary definitions and severity ratings to mental state changes such as depression, euphoria, and intellectual deterioration. In addition, a cut-off age of 40 years was stipulated, in order to avoid the possible complicating factor of menopause. Some patients were also excluded prior to the study onset because of signs of mental illness, as were patients with a duration of MS less than 2 years. The reason for the latter was a desire to include only patients whose symptoms (and diagnosis) were beyond doubt. The many selection criteria produced a biased sample that compromised extrapolating the findings to MS patients in general. Notwithstanding this limitation, results revealed that emotional responses were exaggerated in 11 MS patients (10%) and none of the control subjects. There was no concomitant subjective emotional distress in nine of these patients, suggesting a dissociation between what patients felt and what they expressed. A significant association was noted between the emotional dyscontrol and intellectual decline, similar to Langworthy et al.'s (1941) anecdotal report, but in contrast to Cottrell and

Wilson's observation that such a change was rare (only 2% of their sample was affected). Given this finding, Surridge concluded that emotional dyscontrol was a product of cerebral disease and akin to that seen in pseudobulbar palsy.

In summary, these five studies produced markedly different point prevalence rates ranging from 6.5% to 95%. Arbitrary and inadequate definitions of 'emotional dyscontrol' (used synonymously with pseudobulbar affect, emotional exaggeration, pathological laughing and crying), biased sample selection, and the use of non-standardized interviews of unproven validity and reliability may explain the inconsistent findings.

Definition of pathological laughing and crying

An attempt to bring some diagnostic rigour to a general definition of PLC, irrespective of the underlying neurological disorder, was supplied by Poeck (1969), who distinguished PLC from a number of other symptom complexes. These included emotional lability, which he regarded as episodes of crying (and less frequently laughing) that were excessive, but appropriate to the situation in which it occurred; 'witzelsucht' (facetiousness) and euphoria, associated with a fluctuating and congruent affective tone; and laughing or crying secondary to substance abuse, psychosis or as part of histrionic behaviour. In contrast, PLC was regarded as a distinct syndrome, due to a release of inhibition of the motor component of facial expression. The full syndrome comprised four components: response to non-specific stimuli; absence of an association between affective change and the observed expression; absence of voluntary control of facial expression; and an absence of a corresponding change in mood exceeding the period of laughing or crying. This is the definition that has been adopted in this chapter, although it is acknowledged that such clear subdivisions are not always possible. In practice, a degree of overlap may characterize many presentations begging questions, as yet unresolved, about etiology.

It has been found helpful to conceptualize changes in mood and affect as lying along a continuum. At one end there are patients with a clear diagnosis of major depression who have the subjective complaints of low mood coupled with the objective signs of altered affect. At the other end of the spectrum can be found patients who meet the strict criteria for PLC with loss of control of affect without the subjective compaints of low or elevated mood. Between these two clearly defined syndromes come a number of patients, who display varying degrees of emotional lability, without meeting criteria for either. From a survey of clinic attenders, it is estimated that approximately one in five patients fit this clinical picture (A. Feinstein, unpublished data). These patients to date have slipped through the diagnostic cracks, so to speak, and their clinical distress is often either missed or dismissed as an understandible emotional reaction to having MS. This would seem to do the patients a disservice, because symptoms of emotional lability can by themselves prove disabling. Furthermore, they respond well to treatment. Thus, neatly subdividing emotional and affective change into either a depressive disorder or PLC is often not possible.

Prevalence and neurobehavioural correlates of pathological laughing and crying

Given the failings inherent in earlier studies, accurate demographic, neurological and neurobehavioural correlates of PLC were, until recently, not known. This uncertainty extended to the prevalence of associated psychopathology. While PLC is usually considered distinct from subjective emotional experience such as depression (Minden and Schiffer, 1990), this had not been investigated in a representative sample of MS patients using standardized psychiatric interviews or valid ratings scales and results compared to those from an appropriate control group. In addition, the presence of co-morbid anxiety had yet to be addressed. As for cognitive difficulties, while approximately 40% of MS patients show evidence of intellectual decline (Rao et al., 1991a) that adversely impinges on a wide array of daily activities (Rao et al., 1991b), whether MS patients with PLC were more cognitively impaired than those without had not been ascertained.

Answers to these questions have been supplied by a case control study that overcame many of the methodological shortcomings listed above (Feinstein et al., 1997). A consecutive, outpatient sample of 152 patients with clinically or laboratory definite multiple sclerosis according to the Poser et al. (1983) criteria were screened for the presence of PLC using Poeck's criteria. In addition, subjects were interviewed using the Pathological Laughing and Crying Scale (PLACS)(Robinson et al., 1993), which defines aspects of laughing and crying including duration, relationship to external events, degree of voluntary control, inappropriateness in relation to emotions and extent of subsequent distress.

A group of control subjects with MS, but without PLC, were also drawn from this sample. After neurological examination, they were matched to the PLC group with respect to age, gender, duration of MS, level of disability as defined by the Expanded Disability Status Scale (EDSS), disease course, and premorbid IQ, according to a reading test. Demographic details were recorded on all subjects and controls who subsequently underwent psychiatric and cognitive assessment. Patients with a history of head trauma and substance abuse were excluded, as were those who had undergone previous psychometric assessment, or whose visual acuity precluded testing.

Assessment procedure

Details of a family history of mental illness and premorbid psychiatric problems were noted. Subjects also completed two self-report questionnaires, namely the Hospital Anxiety and Depression Scale (HAD) (Zigmond and Snaith, 1983), developed for assessing patients with physical illness and the 28-item General Health Questionnaire (GHQ) (Goldberg and Hillier, 1979) containing four subscales (anxiety, somatic complaints, social dysfunction and depression) scored the Likert way (0–1–2–3).

Subjects also underwent neurological examination on the day of testing and overall disability assessed with the EDSS. Subscale scores for each of the eight systems were recorded (pyramidal, sensory, brainstem, cerebellar, visual, bladder and bowel, mentation and 'other'). Finally, subjects were screened for general intellectual deficits, with the National Adult Reading Test (NART) (Nelson, 1982) a valid indicator of premorbid intellectual function, and the Wechsler Adult Intelligence Scale-Revised (WAIS-R) (Wechsler, 1981), from which verbal, performance and full-scale intelligence quotients (IQ) were obtained.

Results showed that, of the 152 subjects screened, 15 had PLC, thereby establishing a point prevalence of 9.9%. Comparisons between them and the remainder of the sample revealed no significant age or gender differences. However, the PLC group were more likely to have entered a chronic–progressive disease course and have greater physical disability. The PLC group also had had MS for approximately 2.5 years longer than the remainder of the sample, but this difference did not reach statistical significance. Eleven PLC patients agreed to participate in further psychiatric and cognitive testing, and their results were compared with those from 13 matched control subjects. Six subjects displayed prominent crying, three had difficulties with uncontrollable laughing and two had a mixed picture. The four PLC subjects who refused participation did not differ significantly from the remainder with regard to demographic or disease characteristics.

Demographic and disease-related variables for the PLC (n=11) and control subjects (n=13) are shown in Table 4.1. The mean EDSS score for the PLC group was 6.4 (1.7). There were no differences between PLC patients and controls on any of the EDSS subscales, including brainstem involvement. Given the reported association between the latter and displays of pathological affect (Wilson, 1924) the data were further analysed by dichotomizing the variable 'brainstem involvement' into either 'present' or 'absent' and the PLC patients compared with their controls. This, too, did not produce a significant difference with 7 of the 11 PLC patients (64%) and 7 of the 13 controls (53.8%) having brainstem signs on neurological examination.

Subjects with PLC were not more likely than their controls to have a premorbid or family history of mental illness. The mean PLACS score for the PLC group was significantly higher than the control group's, but they did not

Table 4.1. Demographic and disease characteristics of PLC and control subjects

	PLC group (mean) (sd) ($n=11$)	Control group (mean) (sd) ($n=13$)	χ^2/t-test	df	Sig. (P)
Age	43.7(8.3)	42.5(5.3)	$t=0.5$	22	0.7
Gender (m/f)	4/7	4/9	$\chi^2=0.1$	1	0.8
EDSS	6.4(1.7)	6.2(1.4)	$t=0.3$	22	0.7
pyramidal	4.0(1.2)	3.5(1.3)	$t=0.9$	22	0.4
cerebellar	1.9(1.6)	2.2(1.5)	$t=-0.5$	22	0.6
brain stem	1.5(1.6)	1.1(1.2)	$t=0.8$	22	0.4
sensory	1.4(1.6)	1.4(1.1)	$t=-0.04$	22	1.0
bowel and bladder	1.5(2.2)	1.2(1.5)	$t=0.4$	22	0.7
visual	1.7(1.8)	0.8(1.1)	$t=1.4$	22	0.2
mentation	0.9(0.9)	0.5(0.5)	$t=1.5$	22	0.2
other	0.4(0.5)	0.7(0.6)	$t=-1.4$	22	0.2
Duration of MS (years)	10.4(5.8)	12.2(6.5)	$t=-0.7$	22	0.5
Disease course			$\chi^2=0.02$	1	0.9
Relapsing–remitting	1	1			
Chronic–progressive	10	12			

PLC = Pathological laughing and crying.
EDSS = Expanded Disability Status Scale.
Sig. = Significance.
© 1997, American Medical Association.

differ with respect to HAD anxiety and depression scores (Table 4.2). None of the patients who displayed pathological laughing was judged clinically to be euphoric. The most frequently endorsed GHQ items were in the subscale devoted to social dysfunction (Table 4.2). There was a significant correlation ($r=0.3$; $P=0.001$) between the GHQ social dysfunction score and physical disability (EDSS) for the entire sample ($n=152$). However, patients with PLC did not have higher social dysfunction scores than their control group.

The psychometric results appear in Table 4.3. Premorbid IQ according to the NART for the PLC group was estimated at 110(4.1) and did not differ significantly from the control sample (112.0(5.8)). In both groups, performance IQ on the WAIS-R was more adversely affected than verbal IQ. The PLC patients had lower performance and Full Scale, but not verbal IQ scores.

Analyses of the WAIS-R subscales revealed that the PLC were more impaired on a single verbal subscale, namely Arithmetic and on two of the performance tasks, namely Digit Symbol and Picture Arrangement. A more detailed analysis of the raw Digit Span scores revealed that the PLC and control groups did not differ on Digits Forwards, but significant differences were apparent on Digits Backwards.

Table 4.2. Psychiatric results for PLC and control subjects

	PLC group (n=11) mean(sd)/ median (range)	Control Group (n=13) mean(sd)/ median (range)	t-test/ Mann–Whitney U test	df	Sig. (P)
PLACS score	17.0(10–23)	0(0–12)	$Z=-4.2$		0.00001
HAD: Anxiety score	8.5(3.6)	6.8(4.2)	$t=0.9$	21	0.3
HAD: Depression score	7.1(3.3)	7.5(4.3)	$t=-0.3$	21	0.8
GHQ: Anxiety score	5.7(2.4)	7.3(4.1)	$t=-1.1$	21	0.3
GHQ: Somatic score	4.3(2.5)	6.6(4.2)	$t=-1.5$	21	0.1
GHQ: Social dysfunction score	10.1(3.2)	10.6(3.4)	$t=-0.4$	20	0.7
GHQ: Depression score	4.5(5.2)	4.3(5.6)	$Z=0.0$		1
Total GHQ score	24.6(9.9)	29.1(14.4)	$t=-0.8$	20	0.4

PLACS=Pathological laughing and crying scale score; HAD = Hospital Anxiety and Depression Scale
GHQ = General Health Questionnaire; PLC=pathological laughing and crying
© 1997, American Medical Association.

Summarizing the findings, 10% of a large, consecutive sample of community based patients with MS were found to have PLC, with uncontrollable crying proving more common than laughing. The study was careful to exclude patients whose problem was primarily one of emotional lability. However, the group scores on the PLACS demonstrated that such a clearcut separation was not always possible. The demographic and disease profile to emerge was one without gender predilection, of fairly longstanding disease duration and associated with progressive, significant physical disability, not necessarily of brainstem origin. In conformity with Poeck's notion of PLC, patients did not experience greater subjective emotional distress, but were more intellectually impaired and given this last observation were likely to have more extensive brain involvement than patients without the syndrome (Franklin et al., 1988; Rao et al., 1989; Feinstein et al., 1992).

Etiology

The etiology of PLC is unclear and theories abound (Davison and Kelman, 1939; Ironside, 1956; Dark et al., 1996). Three disparate anatomical levels are thought to play a part; the cortex as controller, the bulbar nuclei as physiological effector and the hypothalamus integrating the two (Black, 1982). Ross

Table 4.3. Psychometric comparisons between PLC and control patients

Test	PLC group (n=11) mean(sd)	Control group (n=13)mean (sd)	t-test/ Mann– Whitney U test	df	Sig. (P)
NART[a]	110.5(4.1)	112.0(5.8)	−0.7	22	0.5
WAIS[b]					
information	9.0(1.7)	10.3(2.6)	−1.4	22	0.2
digit span	10.0(2.8)	11.6(2.6)	−1.5	22	0.2
vocabulary	9.8(1.9)	10.8(2.3)	−1.2	22	0.3
arithmetic	8.0(2.5)	11.0(2.4)	−3.0	22	0.006
comprehension	11.5(1.9)	12.2(2.7)	−0.6	21	0.5
similarities	9.5(1.6)	10.6(1.6)	−1.6	21	0.1
verbal IQ	98.6(9.8)	106.1(12.9)	−1.5	21	0.1
picture completion	7.6(2.4)	9.1(2.1)	−1.6	22	0.1
picture arrangement	6.5(2.3)	9.5(1.8)	−3.5	22	0.002
block design	6.5(2.3)	8.2(1.9)	−2.0	22	0.06
object assembly	5.5(3.2)	7.7(2.1)	−2.0	22	0.07
digit symbol	4.7(1.4)	7.2(2.3)	−3.0	20	0.008
performance IQ	82.6(9.2)	94.6(9.1)	−3.1	21	0.005
full-scale IQ	90.5(8.4)	100.6(10.9)	−2.5	21	0.02

[a]NART=National Adult Reading Test; [b]WAIS=Wechsler Adult Intelligence Scale; PLC=pathological laughing and crying; Sig.=significance.
© 1997, American Medical Association.

and Stewart (1987) have distinguished between pathological affect with and without pseudobulbar palsy. In the former, they acknowledge that the precise anatomical pathways have yet to be ascertained. Bilateral pyramidal motor cortex and pyramidal tract involvement are implicated, but what is less clear are the roles played by the premotor cortex and its descending pathways to the brainstem reticular formation. In PLC without pseudobulbar palsy, unilateral or bilateral lesions affecting the basal forebrain, medial temporal lobe, diencephalon, or tegmentum of the brainstem have been noted.

In addition, pathological affect has also been linked to specific hemisphere dysfunction (Sackheim et al., 1982); pathological laughing with mainly right-sided and pathological crying with predominantly left (dominant) -sided pathology. The associations are not, however, as clearcut. Destructive unilateral lesions may free the contralateral hemisphere, which then drives the emotional response. Similarly, unilateral irritative lesions may have the same effect as contralateral destructive ones. An example is gelastic epilepsy where a left-sided focus produces uncontrollable laughter. Sackheim et al. (1982) also concluded, on the basis of three retrospective studies, that pathological laughing was associated significantly more often with males, and crying with females, and felt this finding could not be solely attributed to ascertainment bias. Rather, the three-way relationship between affect, gender and laterality suggested that males and females differed in terms of dominant and non-dominant hemisphere function when it came to the expression of positive and negative emotions.

Much of the literature devoted to the etiology of pathological affect is either based on retrospectively collected data or confined to theorizing that draws on neuroanatomical and neuropathological knowledge. However, one MS study prospectively investigated the role of the prefrontal cortex in the pathogenesis of PLC. The prefrontal cortex is known to play a prominent part in regulating mood and affect and it was hypothesized that pathology affecting the region could explain the development of PLC (A. Feinstein et al., unpublished data). Eleven MS subjects with PLC were matched to a control group of 13 MS patient without PLC, and prefrontal functional integrity was probed using a measure of conceptual reasoning, namely the Wisconsin Card Sort Test (WCST)(Heaton, 1981), previously shown to be a sensitive marker of frontal lobe involvement in patients with MS. The two groups were then compared on three indices of the Wisconsin Card Sort Test, considered the most sensitive in differentiating patients with frontal from non-frontal pathology, i.e. number of perseverative responses, total errors and number of categories achieved (Arnett et al., 1994).

Neurological data from the study demonstrated that PLC patients were not more likely to have frontal release signs. Similarly, with regard to performance on the WCST, PLC subjects did not differ from their matched controls on the total number of errors or total number of perseverative responses made, or the number of categories completed (Table 4.4). Although there are some dissenting voices (Andersen et al., 1991), performance on the WCST is generally regarded as sensitive to prefrontal pathology and in patients with MS has correlated significantly with the degree of frontal lesion load demonstrated on brain MRI (Arnett et al., 1994). However, it would be premature to conclude from this study that the prefrontal cortex was not involved in PLC. Three distinct prefrontal subcortical circuits have been identified, of which only the dorsolateral prefrontal circuit (DLPFC) subserves conceptual reasoning, the task challenged by the WCST (Cummings, 1993). Thus, pathology in other prefrontal areas, namely the orbitofrontal and anterior cingulate, may yet be implicated in the process. Of the two, the orbitofrontal cortex is the more likely candidate. In Ross and Stewart's (1987) report of pathological crying in two stroke patients, the lesion was confined to a right inferior frontal location in both.

Table 4.4. Psychometric comparisons between patients with (*n*=11) and without (*n*=13) pathological laughing and crying

	PLC group (*n*=11) mean(sd)	Control group (*n*=13) mean(sd)	*t*-test/ Mann– Whitney U test	df	Sig. (*P*)
WAIS: verbal IQ	98.6(9.8)	106.1(12.9)	−1.5	21	0.1
WCST – perseverative errors	17.5(12.2)	18.9(15.2)	−0.3	22	0.8
WCST-total errors	34.6(24.4)	29.7(16.6)	0.6	22	0.6
WCST-categories completed	5.0(1.6)	5.4(1.0)	−0.7	22	0.5

WAIS=Wechsler Adult Intelligence Scale–Revised; WCST=Wisconsin Card Sort Test.

Treatment

PLC can be effectively treated with a number of different drugs at doses that do not cause troublesome side effects. In a double blind, crossover trial, the efficacy of amitriptyline compared to placebo was clearly demonstrated with two-thirds of patients responding significantly to the tricyclic drug (Schiffer et al., 1985). Dosages were, without exception, small, no patient requiring more than 75 mg per day, well below that generally considered optimal for antidepressant effect. In addition, the improvement in pathological affect occurred rapidly (within 48 hours of starting treatment) and independently of any antidepressant effect, adding support to the belief that PLC entails a dissociation between subjective and objective evidence of disturbed affect. Given the low dosages, side effects (dry mouth, drowsiness) were for the most part mild and well tolerated, although in four patients the dosage of amitriptyline had to be reduced. The reason why tricyclic medication proved efficacious is unclear, but may relate to enhancement of dopamine transmission. An increase in the inhibitory neurotransmitter dopamine may therefore rectify a degree of putative cortical–subcortical disinhibition, thought to underpin the syndrome.

Further evidence of dopamine's importance in regulating affect comes from an open trial of levodopa (0.6–1.5 g per day) and amantadine (100 mg per day) in patients with PLC of vascular origin (Udaka et al., 1984). Once again a positive response was observed early in the treatment. No patients were exposed to placebo, but it is unlikely that a placebo response would have exceeded the 40% and 50% of patients who improved on levodopa and amantadine, respectively. The efficacy of treatment was further illustrated by patients relapsing within 1 to 2 weeks of levodopa discontinuation and improving yet again on recommencement of treatment. In addition, bio-chemical evidence implicating abnormal dopamine metabolism was demon-strated by patients with PLC having significantly lower cerebrospinal fluid concentrations of homo-vanillic acid (HVA), but not 5–hydroxyindole acetic acid (%-HIAA). the former being a major metabolite of dopamine.

More recent evidence has demonstrated that fluoxetine, a selective serotonin reuptake inhibitor is also useful in alleviating PLC (Seliger et al., 1992; Sloan et al., 1992). These reports were based on open trials without control groups, patients having either traumatic brain injury or multiple sclerosis. Sample sizes were small (13 and 6, respectively), but in all cases rapid improvement without unpleasant side effects was noted. Although the data on fluoxetine is essentially anecdotal, unlike that for amitriptyline, there appears little to choose between them. Dopamine agonists should be reserved for cases that have not responded to either of the above treatments.

A 43-year-old man with a 10-year history of MS and an EDSS of 4.5 was referred to my clinic after a series of embarrassing events that all pertained to his difficulty in controlling outbursts of laughter. The most recent episode of laughter had led to his eviction from a relative's funeral service and the patient felt deeply distressed by what had occurred. He did not, however, present with features of depression or mania, but instead noted that for the past year his ability to control where, and when, he laughed had steadily lessened. Rather than feeling happy while laugh-ing, he reported feeling embarrassed and ashamed. He had noticed that stressful situations, on occasion, brought out the laughter, although more recently it had started occurring in response to minimal provocation. A diagnosis of pathological crying was made and 25 mg of amitriptyline started, with partial cessation of laughing. The dosage was increased to 50 mg at which point uncontrollable laughing ceased.

Summary

- PLC affects 10% of MS patients.
- Although PLC may overlap with emotional lability, the two terms are not synonymous. Rather, PLC should be regarded as uncontrollable laughing and/or crying without the associated subjective feelings of happiness or sadness, the syndrome usually occurring without any discernable stressor.
- Following on from the above, it is important to emphasize that the presence of PLC does not correlate with either depression or mania.
- PLC is generally associated with disease of long duration, a chronic–

progressive course and moderate physical disability.

- MS patients with PLC are more cognitively impaired than those without, thus indirectly implying a greater brain lesion load. However, no MRI study has specifically addressed this issue.
- The precise pathogenesis of PLC (irrespective of the associated neurological disorder) is not well understood.
- The syndrome often responds quickly to small doses of either amitriptyline, fluoxetine or levodopa and complete symptom resolution may be obtained.

References

Andersen SW, Damasio H, Jones RD, Tranel D. (1991) Wisconsin Card Sorting Test performance as a measure of frontal lobe damage. *Journal of Clinical and Experimental Neuropsychology,* **13**, 909–22.

Arnett PA, Rao SM, Bernardin L, Grafman J, Yetkin FZ, Lobeck L. (1994) Relationship between frontal lobe lesions and Wisconsin Card Sorting Test performance in patients with multiple sclerosis. *Neurology,* **44**, 420–5.

Black DW. (1982) Pathological laughter: a review of the literature. *The Journal of Nervous and Mental Disease,* **170**, 67–71.

Cottrell SS, Wilson SAK. (1926) The affective symptomatology of disseminated sclerosis. *The Journal of Neurology and Psychopathology,* **7**, 1–30.

Cummings JL. (1993) Frontal-subcortical circuits and human behaviour. *Archives of Neurology,* **50**, 873–80.

Dark FL, McGrath JJ, Ron MA. (1996) Pathological laughing and crying. *Australian and New Zealand Journal of Psychiatry,* **30**, 472–9.

Davison C, Kelman H. (1939) Pathologic laughing and crying. *Archives of Neurology and Psychiatry,* **42**, 595–643.

Feinstein A, Feinstein KJ, Gray T, O'Connor P. (1997) The prevalence and neurobehavioural correlates of pathological laughter and crying in multiple sclerosis. *Archives of Neurology,* **54**, 1116–21.

Feinstein A, Kartsounis L, Youl B, Miller D, Ron MA. (1992) Clinically isolated lesions of the type seen in multiple sclerosis: a psychiatric, psychometric and MRI follow-up study. *Journal of Neurology, Neurosurgery and Psychiatry,* **55**, 869–76.

Franklin GM, Heaton RK, Nelson LM, Filley CM, Seibert C. (1988) Correlation of neuropsychological and MRI findings in chronic–progressive multiple sclerosis. *Neurology,* **38**, 1826–9.

Gallagher JP. (1989) Pathologic laughter and crying in ALS: a search for their origin. *Acta Neurologica Scandinavica,* **80**, 114–17.

Goldberg DP, Hillier VF. (1979) A scaled version of the General Health Questionnaire. *Psychological Medicine,* **9**, 139–45.

Heaton RK. (1981) *Wisconsin Card Sort Test Manual.* Odessa, FL: Psychological Association Resources.

Ironside R. (1956) Disorders of laughter due to brain lesions. *Brain,* **79**, 589–609.

Kurtzke JF. (1983) Rating neurologic impairment in multiple sclerosis: an expanded disability status scale (EDSS). *Neurology*, **33**, 1444–52.

Langworthy OR, Kolb LC, Androp S. (1941) Disturbances of behaviour in patients with disseminated sclerosis. *American Journal of Psychiatry*, **98**, 243–9.

Minden SL, Schiffer RB. (1990) Affective disorders in multiple sclerosis. *Archives of Neurology*, **47**, 98–104.

Monteil P, Cohadon F. (1996) Pathological laughing as a symptom of a tentorial edge tumour. *Journal of Neurology, Neurosurgery and Psychiatry*, **60**, 370.

Morris, PLP, Robinson RG, Raphael B. (1993) Emotional lability after stroke. *Australian and New Zealand Journal of Psychiatry*, **27**, 601–5.

Nelson HE. (1982) *National Adult Reading Test: Manual*. Windsor, NFER-Nelson.

Poeck K. (1969) Pathophysiology of emotional disorders associated with brain damage. In *Handbook of Clinical Neurology*, vol. 3, ed. PJ Vinken, GW Bruyn, pp. 343–67. Amsterdam: North Holland Publishing Company.

Poser CM, Paty DW, Scheinberg L. et al. (1983) New diagnostic criteria for multiple sclerosis: Guidelines for research protocols. *Annals of Neurology*, **13**, 227–31.

Pratt RTC. (1951) An investigation of the psychiatric aspects of disseminated sclerosis. *Journal of Neurology, Neurosurgery and Psychiatry*, **14**, 326–35.

Rao SM, Leo GJ, Bernardin L, Unverzagt F. (1991a) Cognitive dysfunction in multiple sclerosis. 1. Frequency, patterns, and prediction. *Neurology*, **41**, 685–91.

Rao SM, Leo GJ, Ellington L, Nauertz T, Bernardin L, Unverzagt F. (1991b) Cognitive dysfunction in multiple sclerosis. 11. Impact on employment and social functioning. *Neurology*, **41**, 692–6.

Rao SM, Leo GJ, Haughton VM, St. Aubin-Flaubert P, Bernardin L. (1989) Correlation of magnetic resonance imaging with neuropsychological testing in multiple sclerosis. *Neurology*, **39**, 161–6.

Robinson RG, Parikh RM, Lipsey JR, Starkstein SE, Price TR. (1993) Pathological laughing and crying following stroke: validation of a measurement scale and double-blind treatment study. *American Journal of Psychiatry*, **150**, 286–93.

Ross ED, Stewart RE. (1987) Pathological display of affect in patients with depression and right frontal brain damage. *Journal of Nervous and Mental Disease*, **175**, 165–72.

Sackheim HA, Greenberg MS, Weinman AL, Gur RC, Hungerbuhler JP, Geschwind N. (1982) Hemisphere asymmetry in the expression of positive and negative emotions. *Archives of Neurology*, **39**, 210–18.

Schiffer RB, Herndon RM, Rudick RA. (1985) Treatment of pathologic laughing and weeping with amitriptyline. *New England Journal of Medicine*, **312**, 1480–2.

Seliger GM, Hornstein A, Flax J, Herbert J, Schroder K. (1992) Fluoxetine improves emotional incontinence. *Brain Injury*, **6**, 267–70.

Sloan RL, Brown KW, Pentland B. (1992) Fluoxetine as a treatment for emotional lability after brain injury. *Brain Injury*, **6**, 315–19.

Starkstein SE, Migliorelli R, Teson A et al. (1995) Prevalence and clinical correlates of pathologic affective display in Alzheimer's disease. *Journal of Neurology, Neurosurgery and Psychiatry*, **59**, 55–60.

Sugar C, Nadell R. (1943) Mental symptoms in multiple sclerosis. *Journal of Nervous and Mental Disease*, **98**, 267–80.

Surridge D. (1969) An investigation into some psychiatric aspects of multiple sclerosis. *British Journal of Psychiatry*, **115**, 749–64.

Udaka F, Yamao S, Nagata H, Nakamura S, Kameyama M. (1984) Pathologic laughing and crying treated with levodopa. *Archives of Neurology*, **41**, 1095–6.

Wechsler D. (1981) *Manual for the Wechsler Adult Intelligence Scale* – revised. New York: Psychological Corporation.

Wilson SAK. (1924) Some problems in neurology. 11. Pathological laughing and crying. *The Journal of Neurology and Psychopathology*, **4**, 1299–333.

Zigmond AS, Snaith RP. (1983) The Hospital Anxiety and Depression Scale. *Acta Psychiatrica Scandinavica*, **67**, 361–70.

Multiple sclerosis and psychosis

Introduction

The association between multiple sclerosis and psychosis is uncommon, which helps explains the paucity of research devoted to the topic. Nevertheless, the relationship is of interest for a number of reasons. These include the possibility that both demyelination and psychosis have a shared, viral pathogenesis, the role of coarse cerebral pathology in the etiology of psychosis, and problems posed by the treatment of psychosis in the neurologically compromised patient.

Psychosis in the context of multiple sclerosis has been termed by the DSM-IV (APA, 1994), 'Psychosis due to a General Medical Condition (PDGMC)' (Table 5.1). The equivalent *International Classification of Disease* (Tenth Edition)(ICD-10)(WHO, 1992) category is one of either 'Organic Hallucinosis', 'Organic Catatonic Disorder', or 'Organic Delusional (schizophrenia-like) Disorder'. This difference in terminology reflects a philosophical divide that separates the taxonomies. Inherent in the DSM approach is the belief that all mental disorders (not just psychotic ones) are 'organic' and that the functional–organic dichotomy is needlessly divisive. The ICD-10, mindful of serving a different constituency (i.e. first- and third-world countries) has retained the word 'organic'. Irrespective of which classification is subscribed to, references on both sides of the Atlantic abound in descriptive terms such as 'schizophrenia-like', 'secondary psychosis' and 'organic psychosis'.

The plethora of terminology also confronts the clinician–researcher with another important dilemma, one that is common to both systems. Is the psychosis due to the MS or is it a chance occurrence? To make a DSM-1V (or ICD-10) diagnosis, there has to be a high index of suspicion that MS has caused the psychosis, which on an individual basis is often difficult. Given that the lifetime prevalence for a psychotic illness such as schizophrenia is approximately 1% and for multiple sclerosis 0.1–0.01% (varying according to lattitude), the two disorders can be expected to appear together by chance every 0.5–1 in 100 000 cases, which approaches the lifetime prevalence of a disorder such as Amytrophic Lateral Sclerosis. Therefore, to make an etiological inference with any degree of certainty, factors supporting face,

Table 5.1 DSM-1V criteria for the diagnostic category, 'Psychosis due to a General Medical Condition'

A.	Prominent hallucinations or delusions
B.	There is evidence from the history, physical examination, or laboratory findings that the disturbance is the direct physiological consequence of a general medical condition.
C.	The disturbance is not better accounted for by another mental disorder.
D.	The disturbance does not occur exclusively during the course of a delirium.

The condition may then be coded according to whether delusions or hallucinations are the most prominent psychotic feature. The general medical condition would also be coded on Axis 111.

Reprinted with permission. © American Psychiatric Association.

descriptive, predictive and construct validity should be present. This applies not only to MS, but to all CNS disorders causally implicated in psychosis. This chapter will review the evidence supporting each of these criteria and also provide guidelines on treatment and assessing outcome.

Literature review

Most reports of MS and psychosis are single case studies with the earliest dating from the nineteenth century. In their comprehensive review of 'schizophrenia-like psychoses associated with organic disorders of the central nervous system (CNS)', Davison and Bagley (1969) devoted a section to demyelinating disease. They reviewed every published report (irrespective of language) of multiple sclerosis that occurred concurrently with a psychotic illness that fulfilled the 1957 WHO criteria for schizophrenia. Given their belief that the presence of coarse cerebral pathology would render some signs and symptoms invalid, they excluded catatonia, autism and change in personality from the WHO guidelines and were left with the following: the presence of an unequivocal disorder of the CNS; the presence at some stage of shallow, incongruous affect, thought disorder, hallucinations and delusions; and the absence, when psychotic, of features suggesting a delirium, dementia, dysmnesic syndrome and affective psychosis. Applying these criteria to their literature review they came across 39 reports, a frequency judged not to exceed chance expectation.

Although Davison and Bagley's conclusions have yet to be empirically validated, some of their findings with respect to other CNS disorders such as epilepsy and basal ganglia disorders have been confirmed (Cummings, 1985; Dewhurst et al., 1969; Popkin and Tucker, 1994). Furthermore, their view that psychosis seldom occurs with MS is cautiously supported by studies investigating the number of MS patients found in large, inpatient psychiatric populations. The percentages from the Massachusetts State Hospital (0.07%), Manhattan State Hospital (0.05%), and Queensland Mental Hospitals (0.06%) are similar and do not exceed chance probability, but may be misleadingly low because of a greater community tolerance for mental disturbance in the presence of MS or alternative admissions to hospitals caring for the physically disabled (Davison and Bagley, 1969).

Summarizing data based largely on anecdotal evidence, there is a consensus that psychosis associated with MS is rare. However, no community-based epidemiological study has been undertaken, which would be the only way to unequivocally establish an accurate estimate of co-morbidity.

Distinguishing characteristics

To make a diagnosis of 'Psychosis due to a General Medical Condition (PDGMC)', the DSM-1V states the physician must first establish the presence of the GMC and then relate the psychosis to it via a physiological mechanism. It is acknowledged there are no infallible guidelines, which accounts for the reported diagnostic uncertainty. Thus, the ICD-10 equivalent of PDGMC has a poor interrater reliability, with a kappa score lower than that for other less 'organic' disorders, thereby reversing an established trend in the classification of mental illness (Lewis, 1994). Despite these difficulties, some pointers to a diagnosis of PDGMC include the following:

Temporal association

A temporal association between the onset, exacerbation and remission of the GMC and the psychotic disturbance should be present. While this makes intuitive sense, an examination of the DSM-1V Sourcebook reveals inconsistent data. The majority of citations pertain to epilepsy and psychosis where, on average, 14 years have elapsed between the onset of seizures and subsequent psychosis (Slater et al., 1963; Feinstein and Ron, 1990). Davison and Bagley's (1969) MS review revealed that, in 36% of cases, the neurological and psychiatric symptoms appeared at approximately the same time. Furthermore, in 61.5% of cases, the psychosis appeared either 2 years before, or after, the onset of neurological symptoms. This temporal association in approximately two-thirds of cases led the authors to conclude that, although psychosis secondary to MS was rare, when it did occur, demyelination was most likely implicated in the pathogenesis. This result was not, however, replicated by Feinstein et al. (1992) in a case control study of ten psychotic MS patients. The mean duration of neurological symptoms before the onset of psychosis was 8.5 years (range 0–19 years). In only one case was the diagnosis of MS made at the time of psychosis onset.

Clinical features

A second consideration recommended by the DSM-IV is the presence of features that would be considered atypical for a primary psychosis, e.g. uncommon clinical features such as olfactory and visual hallucinations. In a study that specifically addressed this issue, Feinstein et al. (1992) examined the case notes of ten psychotic MS patients treated at a tertiary referral centre. Mental state was assessed retrospectively, using the symptom checklist (SCL) derived from the Present State Examination (PSE)(Wing et al., 1974). From the SCL, half the subjects were given a diagnosis of schizophrenia and the other half, an affective psychosis. The commonest symptoms and signs are shown in Table 5.2 and from this it can be seen that lack of insight characterized all the patients' presentations. Persecutory delusions occurred in over two-thirds of cases and were the commonest psychotic feature. Non-specific evidence of psychosis (which included heightened or changed perception, 'minor' hallucinations, e.g. music, noises) were recorded in 60% of patients. Delusions of control (passivity) and delusions with a sexual or fantastic content were present in a third of patients, and delusions of reference noted in one in five patients. The symptom profile was notable for the relative infrequency of well-formed hallucinations. Second person auditory hallucinations were present in 20% of patients as were visual hallucinations. Third person auditory hallucinations (two or more voices commenting on the person) were found in only one case. Thus, delusions in various forms, but particularly with a persecutory content, predominated. The findings lend support to the ICD-10 notion of the psychosis being more akin to an 'organic delusional disorder', with perceptual disturbances less noticeable and of secondary import.

Persecutory delusions were also the most common symptom of psychosis found in other CNS disorders (Slater et al., 1963; Davison and Bagley, 1969; Feinstein and Ron, 1990), with Cummings (1985) noting that relative preservation of cognitive function was necessary for the formation of complex delusional beliefs. Another frequently cited clinical observation of PDGMC, namely the preservation of affective responses also received empirical support (Feinstein et al., 1992). Thus, it would appear that when patients with MS (or any other CNS disorder) become psychotic, the predominant presentation is one of 'positive' psychotic symptoms (delusions, less often hallucinations) with relative preservation of affective responses. The 'negative' or 'defect' state associated with schizophrenia (i.e. apathy, impoverished speech and thought), together with blunted affect is seldom seen. This discriminating feature reflects more than ascertainment bias (see Table 5.1)

Table 5.2 Commonest symptoms and signs (PSE) in a psychotic group of MS patients (*n*=10)

Symptom	%
Lack of insight	100
Persecutory delusions	70
Non-specific evidence of psychosis	60
Irritability	60
Agitation	50
Anxiety	40
Sexual delusions	30
Passivity phenomena	30
Delusions of reference	20
Grandiose delusions	20
Second person auditory hallucinations	20
Visual hallucinations	20
Thought disorder	20
Third person auditory hallucinations	10
Thought broadcast	10

Feinstein et al. (1992).
Reproduced by permission of Royal College of Psychiatry.

for although positive and negative features may frequently coexist in schizophrenia, they seldom do so in PDGMC. Notwithstanding these well-documented group differences that demarcate the clinical picture of MS psychosis from schizophrenia, it needs to be emphasized that, on an individual level, it is frequently difficult to tell the conditions apart. Thus, Slater's view that a patient with psychosis associated with epilepsy is indistinguishable from a patient with schizophrenia applies equally well to the patient with MS who becomes psychotic. It has been the author's experience and that of others (Schmalzbach, 1954; Parker, 1956) that, in MS patients with no obvious neurological deficits, a diagnosis of schizophrenia is readily made. Even in patients with obvious neurological symptoms, the mental state may closely mimic schizophrenia.

Age of presentation

The mean age of first presentation of psychosis in schizophrenic patients is 23 years (Lieberman et al., 1992), which is considerably younger than that for MS patients presenting with psychosis. Thus, Davison and Bagley's review reported a mean age of onset of psychosis a decade older and, in Feinstein et al.'s study, the average age was 36.6 years. A similar picture emerges from studies of other CNS disorders (Slater et al., 1963; Cummings, 1985; Feinstein and

Ron, 1990), and the relatively later age of presentation is therefore further evidence setting PDGMC apart as a distinct diagnostic entity.

Gender ratio

The gender ratio noted in psychotic MS patients differs from that found in either MS or late onset schizophrenia. Thus, Davison and Bagley reported 21 of 39 cases were male, which is at odds with the female to male ratio in MS. Similarly, although the genders are equally represented in schizophrenia (see Lewis, 1992 for a dissenting view), males present earlier than females (Goldstein et al., 1989). As the mean age of onset of psychosis in MS patients is approximately a decade older than in schizophrenia, a preponderance of female psychotic MS patients could be anticipated, which is not the case. These gender discrepancies suggest a central role for demyelination in the pathogenesis of the psychosis.

Etiology

Genetic links

If the psychosis associated with multiple sclerosis was simply the chance co-occurrence of schizophrenia, then one would expect to find increased evidence of schizophrenia in the relatives of the affected proband. Evidence is scanty on this point, but does not support a familial link (Davison and Bagley, 1969). Clinical experience also suggests that premorbid schizoid traits are absent. Once again, it is helpful to look at other CNS disorders for any possible clues to the above questions. Feinstein and Ron (1990) found that 4% of their sample of 65 psychotic patients with heterogenous neurological disorders had a family history of schizophrenia, four times that in the general population. This result is, however, difficult to interpret as the data were not age corrected, the family history method used to assess relatives may have underestimated the true psychiatric morbidity (Andreasen et al., 1983), and the heterogenous nature of the sample meant that some patients with late onset schizophrenia, as opposed to PDGMC, were included, thereby increasing the familial yield. An alternative explanation, however, is that a prevalence rate of 4%, falling between that of the general population and patients with schizophrenia, suggests that the presence of coarse brain pathology may precipitate psychosis in patients with a genetic predisposition.

Viral hypothesis

Stevens (1988) has postulated that similarities in disease course, age of onset, geographical distribution, and immunological response of patients with schizophrenia and multiple sclerosis implies some overlap with respect to pathogenesis. In particular, exposure to a virus at a crucial developmental stage (in utero, childbirth, childhood) may be the common thread linking what are clinically two very different conditions. This viewpoint fits well with current theories of schizophrenia as a neurodevelopmental disorder triggered by insult to the fetal brain (Torrey et al., 1994). Thus, women infected with the influenza virus during the second trimester of pregnancy appear to have an increased risk of producing schizophrenic offspring (O'Callaghan et al., 1991), although some would disagree (Crow and Done, 1992). The hypothesis that an early developmental insult may manifest as illness in adulthood has validity, more so in psychosis, given the weight of published evidence (Castle and Murray, 1991; Murray et al., 1992; O'Connell et al., 1997). Nevertheless, it has also been reported that infection during childhood with the herpes virus may leave some patients prone to develop MS in later life (Sanders et al., 1996), while migration studies have shown that, for those who emigrate after adolescence, the risk of developing MS does not change from that of their country of origin (Dean, 1967).

While theorizing offers intriguing possibilities, the marked differences in clinical presentations between the two disorders outweigh any similarities, making a shared pathogen unlikely.

MRI brain changes

The most compelling evidence linking brain changes in MS to psychosis comes from a case-control MRI study of 10 MS patients with, and 10 without, psychosis (Feinstein et al., 1992), who were matched for age, sex, duration of illness and physical disability. The following PSE (Wing et al., 1974) diagnoses were assigned: schizophrenia (2), schizoaffective psychosis (2), paranoid disorder (1), psychotic depression (1), mania with psychotic features (4).

Subjects and controls underwent contiguous, multislice axial MRI of the brain. All scanning protocols included T_2-weighted images that optimized lesion detection. Patients and controls were scanned over a period of 6 years, during which changes to the MRI scanner and software upgrades ensured better images were obtained. Despite these changes, the imaging protocols and slice thickness were the same in all patient and control groups. It was not, however, possible in one case to match the images for strength of magnetic field. The EDSS and MRI were performed when the patients were psychotic in eight cases. In the remaining two cases, MRI was undertaken 1 and 3 years after the psychotic episode with a normal mental state at the time.

Subjects were compared with controls with respect to site and extent of lesions. MRI analysis was undertaken by a neuroradiologist blind to psychiatric diagnosis. In assessing the MRI, a system derived by Ormerod et al. (1987)

Table 5.3 Mean (sd) MRI lesion scores in psychotic and control patients

	Psychotic patients	Control patients
Total lesion score	32.6(13.6)	27.4(13.8)
Periventricular score	19.3(8.1)	14.0(6.6)
Temporal (bilateral)	8.6(4.3)	6.9(4.4)
Temporal–parietal (bilateral)	12.1(6.2)	9.4(5.6)
Temporal horn R	1.8(0.9)	1.0(0.8)
Temporal horn L	1.7(0.8)	1.0(0.8)
Trigone R	2.2(1.2)	1.7(0.8)
Trigone L	2.3(0.9)	1.5(0.9)
111rd ventricle	0.7(0.5)	0.3(0.5)
Temporal lobe R	0.2(0.6)	0.6(0.9)
Temporal lobe L	0.4(0.8)	1.1(1.5)
Temporal horn+trigone R	4.0(2.1)	2.7(1.6)
Temporal horn+trigone L	4.0(1.6)	2.5(1.4)

No differences were found for frontal lobes/horns, occipital lobes/horns, parietal lobes, internal capsule, basal ganglia, 1Vth ventricle, and cerebellum.
Feinstein et al. (1992).
Reproduced by permission of Royal College of Psychiatry.

was used. The size and presence of lesions were recorded in the following periventricular areas: body of the ventricles; frontal, temporal and occipital horns; trigone; and third and fourth ventricles. These seven areas provided a periventricular score. A further eight areas of brain parenchyma were also examined, namely internal capsule, basal ganglia, frontal, parietal, temporal and occipital lobes; brainstem and cerebellum. The lobes of the cerebrum were defined as including not only cortex, but also underlying white matter. Planes separating lobes were projected from their cortical boundaries to the foramen of Munro or the lateral ventricular trigone, as appropriate. The largest lesion in each particular area was scored using a 4–point scale according to the greatest diameter measured. A total lesion score was obtained by adding scores from all the areas assessed. The percentage of the total lesion score in each particular area was obtained by dividing the score for each area by the total lesion score and multiplying by 100. This was termed the 'percentage score'.

Table 5.3 compares the MRI results of psychotic patients and their matched controls. The psychotic patients had a greater total lesion and periventricular lesion score, but these were not statistically significant. Trends emerged for a higher lesion score in the psychotic group for areas surrounding the temporal horns bilaterally. A similar result was also obtained in the left trigone.

Combining the left temporal horn and adjacent left trigone area scores

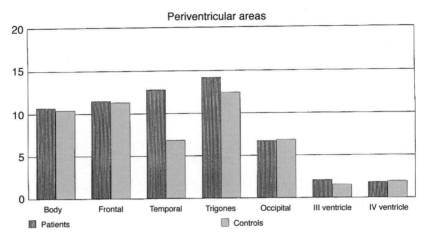

Fig. 5.1.   Percentage lesions score distribution (Feinstein et al., 1992). By permission of the Royal College of Psychiatry.

produced a statistically significant difference between the psychotic and control groups.

A clearer picture of the difference in the distribution of lesion scores between the psychotic and control MS patients was demonstrated by observing what percentage of the total lesion score was present in each particular area. In the controls, the total lesion score was distributed equally between periventricular and other brain areas while in the psychotic patients the periventricular lesion score contributed more than 60% of the total lesion score. This difference was not, however, statistically significant. The most marked differences were present around the temporal horns where the 'percentage score' in the psychotic patients was almost double that of the control group (Fig. 5.1). Thus, not only did the psychotic patients have a greater lesion score, but lesions were differentially distributed in periventricular areas and in particular around the temporal horns of the lateral ventricles. A closer look at the individual patient data demonstrated that, in all but one case control pair, the psychotic patients had a greater temporal horn lesion score than their matched controls (Fig. 5.2).

The various brain areas were also analysed to determine whether the presence or absence of lesions, rather than their size, was the crucial factor, but no differences were found between the groups. In the psychotic group, lesion scores between right and left hemispheres did not differ significantly. In addition, there were no significant correlations between individual psychotic symptoms and MRI lesions.

The study firmly linked psychosis in MS patients to the presence of increased lesion load in temporal areas and, in doing so, confirmed the importance of the region in the pathogenesis of psychosis in general. Enlar-

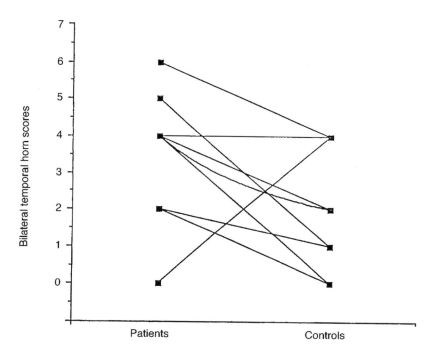

Fig 5.2.   Temporal horn scores (bilateral) for psychotic and non-psychotic subjects.

gement of the left temporal horn at postmortem (Crow et al., 1989) and MRI evidence of reduction in temporal lobe (Suddath et al., 1989) and, in particular, hippocampal volume (Suddath et al., 1990), in patients with schizophrenia attests to this. An association between temporal lobe pathology and PDGMC has also been reported by some (Slater et al., 1963; Davison and Bagley, 1969), but not others (Feinstein and Ron, 1990), although the heterogeneous composition of the latter's sample could explain the discrepant result.

Although the MRI data are compelling, the study had certain shortcomings and left questions unanswered. Limitations pertained to small sample size (indicative of the rarity of an association between MS and psychosis), the possible confounding effects of artefact on MRI quantification, and the scanning of two patients after their psychosis had long resolved. These difficulties were largely offset by a careful case-control design with individual patient-control matching. But, this still left the perplexing question why only certain patients with temporal lobe involvement became psychotic. While the study suggested a 'threshold' lesion volume had to be exceeded before psychosis ensued, this did not invariably apply, as some patients with a large temporal lesion score did not become delusional.

One can therefore posit that, with respect to psychosis, the presence of brain plaques in the temporal lobes is unlikely to fully explain the development of psychosis in all cases. Rather, brain lesions superimposed on a premorbid vulnerability (genetic, developmental, premorbid psychiatric history) seems a more plausible explanation.

Treatment

There are no treatment studies of psychosis associated with MS. Early reports found electroconvulsive treatment (Schmalzbach, 1954) and insulin coma (Parker, 1956) to be ineffective in individual cases. The mainstay of present treatment is neuroleptic medication (Feinstein et al., 1992) and given the often severe nature of the behavioural disturbance, psychiatric hospitalization is often required in the acute stages.

In an analogous situation to that encountered with the floridly manic patient, treatment can present a considerable therapeutic challenge. Experience has taught that MS patients are frequently sensitive to the side effects of neuroleptic medication. Thus, high potency drugs such as the butyrophenones (e.g. haloperidol) which are associated with extrapyramidal side effects (EPS) may further compromise patients mobility and balance, resulting in falls that prove distressing to patients, family and nursing staff. A choice of less potent neuroleptics, such as the phenothiazine groups of compounds lessens the risk of EPS, but anticholinergic difficulties are more prominent, which may aggravate other difficulties such as bladder and bowel control and impaired vision. The associated dry mouth may add to dysarthric difficulties. All neuroleptic medication, irrespective of class, can produce excessive sedation which may similarly affect already impaired coordination and balance.

With these difficulties in mind, small doses of neuroleptic medication are recommended. Such an approach is supported by the results of a functional imaging study in schizophrenia which has shown that 2 mg of haloperidol blocks up to three-quarters of dopamine D2 receptors, thereby exerting substantial clinical improvement without troubling side effects (Kapur et al., 1996). The authors have recommended treating psychotic patients with doses of haloperidol that do not exceed 2 to 4 mg per day. Applying these guidelines to psychotic MS patients makes clinical and pharmacological sense, although it has been my experience that doses even this small may exacerbate some patients' neurological difficulties.

Newer antipsychotic drugs offer less prominent side effects. Furmaga et al. (1995) have reported that risperidone was helpful in ten patients with PDGMC, who had not previously responded to a conventional neuroleptic. Clozapine, which has the advantage of few EPS problems, has a proven efficacy in patients with movement disorders who become psychotic (Chacko et al., 1995) and is an alternative to risperidone. Weekly blood checks are required to monitor for the development of agranulocytosis that affects 1% of patients on treatment. Postural hypotension early in the treatment carries with it the risk of falls in patients who are neurologically impaired, but this difficulty is transient and lessens significantly after a few weeks of treatment. Seizures are another risk factor at higher doses (in excess of 600 mg per day), but such doses are rarely needed. Olanzapine, a thiobenzodiazepine, recently introduced to the North American market, potentially offers the benefits of clozapine, without agranulocytosis. It also has the advantage of a convenient once a day dose (recommended dose of 10 mg per day) which can be started immediately. Its efficacy in psychotic MS patients has not yet been ascertained.

Should behavioural control still be required despite adequate antipsychotic dosage, benzodiazepines may be added. Lorazepam has the advantage of being given either via the oral or intramuscular route. Oral dosages rarely exceed 8 mg per day, and the clinician should bear in mind that the intramuscular dose is equivalent to 2–21 times the oral dose, because it avoids the first pass metabolism.

Some of these points are illustrated by the following case history.

A 38-year-old, divorced, unemployed woman with a 4-year history of MS (EDSS of 2.0) was brought by her mother to see me, as the family were concerned about her behaviour and by some of the things she was saying. There was no family history of mental illness and the patient had been well until the age of 35 years when, after a bout of optic neuritis, followed almost immediately by a loss of sensation affecting her right arm, a diagnosis of MS was made. The patient made a good neurological recovery, but 3 years later, after a brief episode of optic neuritis, began speaking of the special relationship she had with members of the English Royal family. She maintained the Queen was able to place thoughts in her head and control what she was thinking, saying and doing. In addition, she openly spoke of hearing voices belonging to members of the Royal family talking about her and commenting, in an unpleasant way, on how she was dressed and the standard of her clothing.

By the time I was consulted, she had been symptomatic for 3 months. In addition to confirming the presence of grandiose delusions and passivity phenomena (delusions of control), I was also able to witness the patient responding verbally to her auditory hallucinations which were in the nature of two voices discussing her in the third person (a Schneiderian first-rank symptom of schizophrenia). Her mood was normal. A diagnosis of 'psychosis due to a general medical condition (i.e. MS)' was made and outpatient treatment in the form of haloperidol 1 mg b.i.d. started. Compliance with medication was ensured by the patient's mother, yet the patient's mental state had not changed when she was seen again 1 month later. The dosage of haloperidol was therefore increased to 2 mg b.i.d.

with a cessation in the auditory hallucinations, but at the cost of bradykinesia and akathisia.

Faced with a choice of treating the bradykinesia with anticholinergic medication and the akathisia with a ß-blocker such as propranalol, or alternatively switching neuroleptic drugs to one of the newer compounds, the latter was decided on. Haloperidol was stopped and risperidone 0.5 mg b.i.d. started. The medication was well tolerated and after a week the dosage increased to 1 mg b.i.d. and 2 weeks later to 1.5 mg b.i.d., at which point auditory hallucinations had stopped and delusional beliefs had reduced in intensity to the point of becoming over-valued ideas. There was no evidence of neuroleptic-induced side effects at this dosage. The patient remained on risperidone for a period of 6 months and then, no longer psychotic, asked to come off treatment. The risperidone was tapered over the course of a month and then stopped. A year later, her mental state remains essentially normal and the remission in her MS continues.

Given the good response to risperidone, why was this drug not prescribed as a first choice? It is my opinion that the newer antipsychotic drugs should, indeed, be the first choice in treatment, but at present, prescribing practice as mandated by state reimbursement schemes insist that the newer (and considerably more expensive) antipsychotic drugs can only be dispensed once patients have a proven, documented inability to tolerate an older, conventional (and considerably cheaper) drug. The adverse reactions can include parkinsonian symptoms, akathisia, dystonic reactions and the tardive spectrum of movement disorders.

Outcome

Earlier literature, much of it predating the appearance of neuroleptic medication in the early 1950s, reported psychotic MS patients either recovered spontaneously, progressed from psychosis to dementia or ran a relapsing–remitting course with respect to psychosis and MS that ultimately went on to dementia. More recent data demonstrate that neuroleptic medication has substantially altered this outlook. Of ten psychotic patients followed for approximately 6 years, the median duration of their first psychotic episode was 5 weeks (range 1 to 72 weeks). Six (60%) of the patients did not experience another psychotic episode, three patients had one further relapse, and a single patient multiple recurrences. Overall, the psychosis remitted in 90% of cases, with a chronic, paranoid psychosis ensuing in a single patient. In general, patients did not require long-term oral or depot neuroleptic use. If a relapse occurred, short-term neuroleptic medication was reintroduced and subsequently discontinued after improvement in the mental state (Feinstein et al., 1992).

The outcome is thus better than in schizophrenia and is similar to other neurological disorders giving rise to PDGMC (Slater et al., 1963; Feinstein and Ron, 1990). The outcome data also overlap with that in late onset schizophrenia (Harris and Jeste, 1988), suggesting that age is an important modifier of outcome. Although Feinstein et al.'s (1992) duration of follow-up did not exceed 6 years, this result may also accurately reflect long-term outcome. Follow-up of schizophrenic patients has shown that decline is most rapid within the first 5 years of initial presentation, after which the condition tends to plateau (Keith and Mathews, 1994).

Summary

- Psychosis associated with MS is a rare occurrence and probably does not exceed chance expectation.
- A case control study has demonstrated that psychotic MS patients are more likely to have plaques involving the temporal horn areas bilaterally.
- There are data to suggest that MS-related psychosis is distinct from schizophrenia, based on a later age of presentation, preservation of affective response, quicker resolution of symptoms, fewer psychotic relapses, better response to treatment and more favourable outcome.
- Neuroleptic drugs such as clozapine and risperidone, in small doses, are the treatment of choice, although reports of their efficacy are anecdotal. Benzodiazepines may be used as an adjunct for sedation.

References

American Psychiatric Association. (1994) *Diagnostic and Statistical Manual of the American Psychiatric Association*, Fourth Edition. Washington DC: American Psychiatric Press.

Andreasen NC, Rice J, Endicott J, Reich T, Coryell W. (1983) The family history approach to diagnosis: how useful is it? *Archives of General Psychiatry*, **43**, 421–9.

Castle D, Murray RM. (1991) The neurodevelopmental basis of sex differences in schizophrenia. *Psychological Medicine*, **21**, 565–75.

Chako RC, Hurley RA, Harper RG, Jankovic J, Cardoso F. (1995) Clozapine for acute and maintenance treatment of psychosis in Parkinson's disease. *Journal of Neuropsychiatry and Clinical Neurosciences*, **7**, 471–5.

Crow TJ, Done DJ. (1992) Prenatal exposure to influenza does not cause schizophrenia. *British Journal of Psychiatry*, **161**, 390–3.

Crow TJ, Ball J, Bloom SR et al. (1989) Schizophrenia as an anomaly of development of cerebral asymmetry: a post mortem study and a proposal concerning the genetic basis of the disease. *Archives of General Psychiatry*, **46**, 1145–50.

Cummings JL. (1985) Organic delusions: phenomenology, anatomical correlations and review. *British Journal of Psychiatry*, **146**, 184–97.

Davison K, Bagley CR. (1969) Schizophrenia-like psychoses associated with organic disorders of the central nervous system. A review of the literature. In *Current Problems in Neuropsychiatry*, ed. RN Herrington, pp. 113–84. Ashford, Kent: Hedley.

Dean G. (1967) Annual incidence, prevalence and morbidity of multiple sclerosis in white South African-born and in white immigrants to South Africa. *British Medical Journal*, **2**, 724–30.

Dewhurst K, Oliver J, Trick KLK, McKnight AL. (1969) Neuropsychiatric aspects of Huntington's disease. *Confinia Neurologica*, **31**, 258.

Feinstein A, Ron MA. (1990) Psychosis associated with demonstrable brain disease. *Psychological Medicine*, **20**, 793–803.

Feinstein A, du Boulay, G, Ron MA. (1992) Psychotic illness in multiple sclerosis. A clinical and magnetic resonance imaging study. *British Journal of Psychiatry*, **161**, 680–5.

Furmaga KM, DeLeon O, Sinha S, Jobe T, Gaviria M. (1995) Risperidone response in refractory psychosis due to a general medical condition. *Journal of Neuropsychiatry and Clinical Neurosciences*, **7**, 417 (abstract).

Goldstein JM , Tsuang MT, Faraone SV. (1989) Gender and schizophrenia: implications for understanding the heterogeneity of the illness. *Psychiatry Research*, **28**, 243–53.

Harris MJ, Jeste D. (1988) Late onset schizophrenia: an overview. *Schizophrenia Bulletin*, **14**, 39–55.

Kapur S, Remington G, Jones C et al. (1996) High levels of dopamine D_2 receptor occupancy with low dose haloperidol treatment: a PET study. *American Journal of Psychiatry*, **153**, 948–50.

Keith SJ, Mathews SM. (1994) The diagnosis of schizophrenia: a review of onset and duration issues. In *DSM-1V Sourcebook*, ed. T. Widiger, A. Francis, H. Pincus et al, pp. 393–418. Washington DC: American Psychiatric Press.

Lewis S. (1992) Sex and schizophrenia: vive la difference. *British Journal of Psychiatry*, **161**, 445–50.

Lewis, S. W. (1994) ICD-10: a neuropsychiatric nightmare. *British Journal of Psychiatry*, **164**, 157–8.

Lieberman JA, Alvir A, Woerner M et al. (1992) Prospective study of psychopathology in first episode schizophrenia at Hillside Hospital. *Schizophrenia Bulletin*, **18**, 351–71.

Murray RM, O'Callaghan E, Castle DJ, Lewis SW. (1992) A neurodevelopmental approach to the classification of schizophrenia. *Schizophrenia Bulletin*, **18**, 319–32.

O'Callaghan E, Sham P, Takei N, Glover G, Murray RM. (1991) Schizophrenia after exposure to 1957 A2 influenza epidemic. *Lancet*, **1**, 1248–50.

O'Connell P, Woodruff PWR, Wright I, Jones P, Murray RM. (1997) Developmental insanity or dementia praecox: was the wrong concept adopted? *Schizophrenia Research*, **23**, 97–106.

Ormerod IEC, Miller DH, McDonald WI et al. (1987) The role of NMR imaging in the assessment of multiple sclerosis and isolated neurological lesions. *Brain*, **110**, 1579–616.

Parker N. (1956) Disseminated sclerosis presenting as schizophrenia. *Medical Journal of Australia*, **1**, 405–7.

Popkin MK, Tucker GJ. (1994) Mental disorders due to a general medical condition and substance-induced disorders. Mood, anxiety, psychotic, catatonic and personality disorders. In *DSM-1V Sourcebook*, ed. TA Widiger, AJ Frances, HA Pincus et al. ch. 17, pp. 243–76. Washington DC: American Psychiatric Association.

Sanders VJ, Waddell AE, Felisan SL, Li X, Conrad AJ, Tourtellotte WW. (1996) Herpes simplex virus in postmortem multiple sclerosis brain tissue. *Archives of Neurology*, **53**, 125–33.

Schmalzbach O. (1954) Disseminated sclerosis in schizophrenia. *Medical Journal of Australia*, **1**, 451–2.

Slater E, Beard AW, Glithero E. (1963) The schizophrenia-like psychoses of epilepsy. *British Journal of Psychiatry*, **109**, 95–150.

Stevens JR. (1988) Schizophrenia and multiple sclerosis. *Schizophrenia Bulletin*, **14**, 231–41.

Suddath RL, Casanova MF, Goldberg TE, Daniel DG, Kelsoe JR., Weinberger DR. (1989) Temporal lobe pathology in schizophrenia: a quantitative magnetic resonance imaging study. *American Journal of Psychiatry*, **146**, 464–72.

Suddath RL, Christison GW, Torrey EF, Casanova MF, Wenberger DR. (1990) Anatomical abnormalities in the brains of monozygotic twins discordant for schizophrenia. *New England Journal of Medicine*, **322**, 789–94.

Torrey EF, Taylor E, Bracha HS et al. (1994) Prenatal origin of schizophrenia in a subgroup of discordant monozygotic twins. *Schizophrenia Bulletin*, **20**, 423–32.

Wing JK, Cooper JE., Sartorius N. (1974) *The Measurement and Classification of Psychiatric Symptoms. An Instruction Manual for the Present State Examination and CATEGO Programme.* Cambridge: Cambridge University Press.

World Health Organization (1992) *The International Classification of Diseases*, 10th Edition. Geneva: WHO.

6

Cognitive impairment in multiple sclerosis

That most perceptive of behavioural neurologists, Charcot (1877) observed that MS patients may show 'marked enfeeblement of the memory, conceptions are formed slowly and intellectual and emotional faculties are blunted in their totality'. Despite this early recognition of potential cognitive difficulties in MS patients, for the greater part of this century clinicians have held to the belief that cognitive difficulties were seldom part of the clinical picture in MS, and if present, generally confined to patients with severe physical disability. Thus, Kurtzke (1970), on the basis of a clinical examination, estimated that cognitive difficulties affected less than 5% of patients. Even more striking were the conclusions of Cottrell and Wilson's (1926) influential study of 100 MS patients seen in a tertiary referral centre. Noting intellectual decline in only two cases, the authors considered the problem 'minimal and negligible'. Although this is now known not to be the case, one reason for clinicians missing the diagnosis can be traced to the nature of cognitive impairment in a subcortical disease such as MS, where the more readily discernable deficits such as agnosia, apraxia and language difficulties, characteristic of cortical dementias, are for the most part absent.

With the advent of magnetic resonance imaging in the early 1980s, clinicians and researchers were able to visualize the brain's white matter changes with a new-found clarity. The ability to detect cerebral lesions in vivo was the impetus for researchers to look for clinical correlates, be they neurological or related to mentation, and MS became attractive to researchers as the prototypical subcortical, white matter dementing process. But, first the prevalence and nature of cognitive changes had to be re-examined, using the more sensitive methods of neuropsychological testing. The result was an outpouring of research data documenting cognitive dysfunction in MS. Within less than 20 years, Kurtzke's figure of less than 5% was revealed as a gross underestimate. When in 1990, the cognitive Function Study Group of the National Multiple Sclerosis Society (Peyser et al., 1990) published their guidelines for neuropsychological research in MS, their review of the literature estimated that 54% to 65% of MS patients were cognitively impaired.

However, it was also becoming clear that the pendulum may have swung too far in the opposite direction. MS patients are a heterogenous group, comprising individuals whose illness differs with respect to duration of symptoms, physical disability, frequency of disease exacerbations, disease course and site of lesions. Furthermore, the studies that had consistently found cognitive impairment in well over half the sample contained an inbuilt bias, for they utilized clinic attenders, a group who were potentially more severely affected by their disease than a community-based sample. New studies were therefore needed, using a more representative sample selection and controlling for a host of disease and demographic-related variables.

Prevalence of cognitive impairment

Two studies followed this approach and their results are comparable. Rao et al. (1991a) initially approached 730 community-based MS patients via mail. Approximately 10% refused participation, while a number of other factors (uncertainties over diagnosis, previous psychometric assessment, a history of alcohol or drug abuse or a concomitant neurological disorder, patient deceased) reduced the number of subjects to 100. All subjects had a neurological examination and information on disease course, physical disability, duration of illness from symptom onset and from diagnosis, and current medications obtained. One hundred healthy control subjects were matched to the MS group with respect to age, gender and number of years of education. Both groups then completed a neuropsychological battery of 31 tests that included the Mini-Mental State Examination (Folstein et al., 1975) and tests of verbal intelligence, immediate, recent and remote memory, abstract reasoning, attention and concentration, language and visuospatial perception. Cognitive function was rated as impaired if scores fell below the fifth percentile scores of the normal control subjects.

Compared to healthy controls, the results revealed that MS patients failed significantly more tests (mean=4.64 (sd=4.9) vs. mean 1.13 (sd=1.8)). If subjects failed on four or more cognitive indices, they were deemed cognitively impaired, which was the case in 48 MS patients and 5 controls. The false positive rate (i.e. 5) was subtracted from the true positive rate, leaving a frequency of cognitive impairment of 43%.

This result has been replicated by McIntosh-Michaelis et al. (1991), also in a community-based sample of 147 patients with MS. A group of 34 patients with rheumatoid arthritis (RA) were included for comparison as the authors wanted to control for any possible effects of depression on psychometric performance. The two groups were matched for gender and number of years of schooling, but not age (the RA patients were significantly older). All subjects completed a neuropsychological battery that included the Rivermead Behavioural Memory Test (RBMT), the Modified Wisconsin Card Sort Test (MWCST), the Controlled Oral Word Association Test (COWAT) and two tests of general intellectual ability, namely the verbal subscale of the

Wechsler Adult Intelligence Scale-Revised (WAIS-R) and the Raven's Standard Progressive Matrices, the latter chosen instead of the performance subscale of the WAIS-R to reduce the effects of sensorimotor impairment on performance. Cognitive impairment was defined as deficits on three measures, i.e. verbal and performance IQ and any one of the RBMT, COWAT, and the MWCST. The result was that 46% of MS patients and 12% of the RA patients were found to be impaired.

The above studies also concurred on the relationship between cognitive impairment and other disease-related variables. Thus, both noted a weak association between cognitive impairment and physical disability as measured by the Expanded Disability Status Scale (EDSS), but failed to find a clear association with disease duration, although McIntosh-Michaelis et al. (1991) noted that memory impairment alone was related to a disease duration of greater than 10 years. An indication of how important sample selection may prove in determining the prevalence of cognitive dysfunction is shown in a study by van den Burg et al. (1987). Although also utilizing a community-based sample drawn from a well-defined epidemiological catchment area in Holland, the authors restricted sample selection to patients with an EDSS not exceeding 4. In addition, the distribution of subjects over the EDSS range of 1 to 4 was kept uniform. Selection was further restricted by excluding patients who had experienced a disease exacerbation within the previous 2 months. With the emphasis on targeting a less disabled subgroup of patients, and comparing neuropsychological performance to an age, sex and education matched group of healthy controls, the number of MS patients found to be cognitively impaired was less than half those of the Rao and McIntosh-Michaelis' samples.

The results of these community-based neuropsychological studies may be contrasted with the results of *clinically* derived estimates from similar populations. Kahana et al.'s (1971) and Shepherd's (1979) estimates of 7% and 25%, respectively, illustrate the reduced sensitivity of clinical as opposed to neuropsychological methods.

A more detailed review of the salient aspects of cognition in MS follows.

General intelligence

As a group, MS patients have IQs within the normal range when examined cross-sectionally and when premorbid IQ is inferred from educational and employment records. However, this broad generalization risks overlooking significant, albeit mild degrees of deterioration. Canter (1951) administered the Army General Classification Test to 23 men who had developed MS after joining the military. The men had all completed the same test prior to enrolment and Canter therefore had the unique opportunity of comparing premorbid performance with that post-MS onset. The test–retest duration was up to 4 years and a significant drop of 13.5 IQ points was noted. This remains the only study that can directly call on a measure of premorbid intellect as a means of comparison. An alternative approach has been to assess premorbid IQ with a reading test such as the National Adult Reading Test (NART)(Nelson, 1982) and then compare this estimate with a current measure of IQ as determined by the Wechsler Adult Intelligence Scale (WAIS)(Wechsler, 1955). Subtracting the WAIS from the NART score supplies a measure of change in intellect and using this method, Ron et al. (1991) found a significant decline in MS patients compared with a group of disabled controls subjects who had neurological disorders sparing the brain. When interpreting these findings, it should be remembered that scores on the Wechsler performance subscale generally are 7–14 points lower than the verbal subscale (Rao et al., 1987), which may be more a reflection of sensorimotor than of visuospatial difficulties.

The results of these two studies have, however, largely been negated by a host of contrary findings. Longitudinal research (see Chapter 7) has shown that decline in IQ may be, for the most part, confined to scores on performance subscales (Canter, 1951) with verbal scores either remaining unchanged or improving (Fink and Houser, 1966). Furthermore, studies using the WAIS have failed to report differences between MS patients and a variety of control groups. Jambor (1969) undertook a four-way comparison between MS patients, healthy controls, psychiatric patients (diagnoses unspecified) and disabled patients without CNS involvement (e.g. muscular dystrophy) and reported similar intergroup scores on a shortened version of the verbal subscale. Goldstein and Shelly (1974), while replicating this finding with respect to psychiatric patients (schizophrenia, depression), also reported that non-MS brain-damaged patients had similar scores. The greatest difficulties experienced by the MS patients were with tests reliant on motor performance. Reitan et al. (1971), while recognizing this fact, also noted differences in verbal IQ between MS patients and age and education matched healthy controls. However, the mean verbal IQ in their MS group was still in the upper normal range, and it was unclear whether this represented a decline from premorbid functioning.

Before concluding that decline in intelligence is primarily limited to performance IQ, two points need emphasizing. First, there is considerable individual variability in the IQ scores of MS patients, which is reflective of the variability that characterizes their cognitive abilities in general. Focusing on group scores may therefore obscure significant declines in individual patients. Secondly, there are more subtle indications of impairment on one of the verbal subscales. The digit-span is a composite score of recalling digits forwards and backwards and MS patients as a group perform normally on this test. However, when the forward and backward components are analysed separately, deficits that are masked by the total score may become apparent on the backwards recall (Rao et al., 1991a; Feinstein et al., 1997).

Memory and multiple sclerosis

A substantial number of MS patients have memory impairment. Staples and Lincoln (1979) reported a figure of 60% in a sample with advanced disease, while Rao et al. (1984), confining their investigation to patients with a chronic-progressive disease course, found 21% with moderate to severe memory impairment, 43% with mild deficits and 36% with no evidence of memory loss. These results are supported by community-based studies with a more representative patient sample. Thus, Rao et al. (1991a) noted that a quarter to a third of 100 community-based MS patients performed poorly on tests of recent memory, a figure replicated by McIntosh-Michaelis et al. (1991). In a study that randomly selected patients from the community and an inpatient neurological service, 30% of MS patients were severely memory impaired, 30% had moderate impairment while only 40% had little or no impairment (Minden et al., 1990). Given the frequency of memory impairment in MS, this area has been more extensively studied that any other aspect of cognition, but before reviewing the findings, some theoretical and semantic clarifications are needed.

There is controversy amongst neuropsychologists when it comes to conceptualizing memory (Squire, 1987; Schacter and Tulving, 1994). The remit of this chapter is not, however, to review the respective merits of each theory, but rather to emphasize that memory is a function of many different systems which may be affected to various degrees in multiple sclerosis. Unfortunately, the potential for confusion is not helped by a plethora of terms that refer to the same phenomenon. Nevertheless, an useful diagrammatic approach to understanding memory is provided by Hodges (1994) (Fig. 6.1) and the review that follows will adhere to this outline, although it is acknowledged that not all aspects of memory fit into the schema.

Implicit memory (procedural memory)

This refers to memory that is not reliant on conscious recall and encompasses motor skills, conditioning and priming. It differs from explicit (or declarative) memory that is accessed through conscious effort. There is a consensus that MS patients perform normally on tests of motor skill (Beatty et al., 1990a) and priming (stem completion)(Beatty and Monson, 1990). Similarly, Grafman et al. (1991) found that MS patients performed normally on tasks that required automatic, but not effortful processing. Noting similarities between automatic processing (frequency and modality monitoring) and

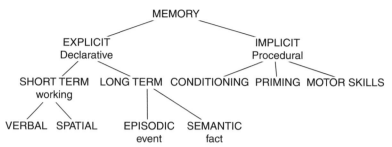

Fig. 6.1   Schematic representation of memory systems.

implicit memory, the authors hypothesised that such processes may require predominantly cortical structures, unlike explicit memory which requires effort and may be more closely related to the functional integrity of subcortical structures, and thus more likely to be affected in MS.

Short-term memory (working memory, immediate memory, primary memory)

This system is responsible for the immediate recall of small amounts of verbal and non-verbal (spatial) information. Short-term memory may be divided into two broad subcomponents, namely the phonological (or articulatory loop) and the visuo-spatial sketchpad. The former is responsible for the recollection of words, numbers and melodies, while the latter is confined to the recall of spatial information. Both components are controlled by a central executive that regulates the distribution of limited attentional resources and controls cognitive processing when novel tasks are presented or existing habits need to be overridden (Baddeley, 1986). Earlier theory, which held that short-term memory had to be intact for the information to reach long-term memory, is now thought to be an oversimplification. The system probably functions independently of, but in parallel with, long-term memory.

Short-term memory may be assessed in a number of different ways, i.e. the amount of information held in store (digit-span), the rate of scanning the information in short-term storage, and the ability to access the memory store in the presence of verbal distracters.

The amount of information held in a short-term memory store (digit-span) is either normal (Jambor, 1969; Rao et al., 1984; Heaton et al., 1985) or mildly impaired (Lyon-Caen et al., 1986; Huber et al., 1987; Fischer, 1988; Kujala et al. 1996) in relation to healthy subjects. Both Rao et al. (1991a) and Feinstein et al. (1997) have distinguished between the forwards and backwards components of the test and found MS patients to be impaired on the latter, more complex task. When it comes to assessing the rate of scanning information held in the short-term memory store, results have been inconsistent with some (Rao et al., 1989a; 1991a), but not others (Litvan et al., 1988a) reporting abnormalities in reaction times. In general, MS patients have retained the ability to store information in short-term memory and access it despite the presence of distracters, i.e. the Brown Petersen task (Litvan et al. 1988b; Beatty et al., 1989a; Rao et al., 1989b; 1991a), although there is a suggestion that performances may become impaired in the presence of disease exacerbations (Grant et al., 1984) or if the disease course becomes chronic–progressive (Beatty et al., 1988).

In addition, D'Esposito et al. (1996) have suggested that working memory impairments in MS patients may relate to dysfunction within the central executive system. MS patients displayed more deficits than healthy controls on a primary task during a dual task paradigm, particularly when the complexity of the secondary task was increased. This result, which correlated with performance on another test probing information processing speed (i.e. the PASAT) may be interpreted as an inability of the central executive to provide sufficient attentional resources required to process multiple tasks simultaneously.

Whether deficits in short-term memory are, in part, responsible for long-term memory deficits is unclear, although Litvan et al. (1988b), posit an association via a breakdown in the phonological loop. However, no attempt has been made to replicate their findings, and some inconsistencies in their data have led Grafman et al. (1990) to question their significance.

Long-term (secondary) memory

Long-term memory refers to memory for information that exceeds the capacity for primary memory. In turn, this can be subdivided into two systems, that pertaining to personal (biographical) events and their temporal sequence, referred to as episodic memory and memory containing a store of representational knowledge of facts and concepts, called semantic memory.

It is in relation to secondary memory that deficits in MS patients are most apparent. This finding, which has been demonstrated with different paradigms, applies equally to verbal and non-verbal memory (Staples and Lincoln, 1979; Grant et al., 1984; Rao et al., 1984, 1991a; Caine et al., 1986; Beatty et al., 1988).

Memory deficits are more readily discernable on tests of recall as opposed to recognition (Rao, 1986). The discrepancy between recall and recognition suggests the problem is mainly one of *retrieval* and not the encoding of new information. Further evidence of retrieval problems is illustrated by difficulties MS patients have with verbal fluency (Beatty et al., 1988; Rao et al., 1991a), indicative of a retrograde memory loss. More recently, evidence suggesting difficulties with memory *acquisition* have been reported. Although the ability to learn with repeated presentation of stimuli (i.e. multitrial learning) may vary considerably between MS patients, both Rao et al. (1984) and Fischer et al. (1992) were able to separate patients according to three patterns of performance; normal rate of learning, impairment on the first trial with a subsequent normal rate of learning and impaired initial and subsequent learning. DeLucca et al. (1994) demonstrated that MS patients required significantly more trials to initially learn a task, relative to healthy controls, but once learnt, did not differ from healthy controls in delayed recall of verbal material, nor in recognition memory performance. The authors make the point that studies stating memory difficulties are predominantly those of retrieval, have often not controlled for the effects of defective acquisition. Comprehensive reviews of the neuropsychological literature pertaining to memory deficits in MS largely echo these conclusions (Wishart and Sharpe 1997; Thornton and Raz, 1997). In all but a few patients, the heterogeneity of findings therefore makes it likely both acquisition and retrieval difficulties are present (Beatty, 1993; Beatty et al., 1996).

Some researchers have approached memory difficulties from another perspective, focusing not on how much information can be remembered, but rather on strategies employed for remembering, in particular, the ability of MS patients to attach meaning to what they learn, i.e. semantically encode and retrieve verbal material. If MS patients are able to learn and retain new information by a process of attaching meaning, this would offer avenues for remediation. An earlier study (Carroll et al., 1984) demonstrated that semantic processing did aid recall, but the process itself had the potential to confuse MS patients. These findings were extended by Goldstein et al. (1992) who found that semantic processing that involved gist recall (i.e. memory for the more important aspects of the information) was intact in MS patients. Thus, while MS patients recalled fewer items than healthy control subjects, the items they remembered were of greater importance. Given that gist recall may be affected by the speed with which information processing takes place, it remains to be seen whether MS patients are able to transfer this ability from the laboratory to the natural environment.

Another aspect to secondary memory, namely remote memory, has been studied in MS patients by challenging their recall and recognition of famous faces and events from the past. Deficits on remote memory would also support a problem with retrieval, but here results have been equivocal, with some (Beatty et al., 1988, 1989a; Beatty and Monson, 1991), but not others (Rao et al., 1991a) noting abnormalities.

Metamemory

Finally, the ability of MS patients to accurately appraise their own memory (termed metamemory), particularly with respect to newly acquired information, is also compromised (Beatty and Monson, 1991). This observation, which cannot be related to the mood state of the patient, is important clinically, for it implies that patients' self-reports about memory are likely to be inaccurate. Metamemory may be, in part, a function of the prefrontal cortex. Taylor (1990) compared objective evidence of cognitive ability (neuropsychological test performance) with patients' subjective assessments of their cognitive function and reported discrepancies. The association was closer when informants' ratings of the subjects' impairment were compared with the objective evidence. Consistent with Beatty and Monson's (1991) observation of metamemory as a function of frontal integrity, Taylor noted that the greatest discrepancies in his sample occurred in patients who did poorly on frontal lobe tests.

In a related study Sullivan et al. (1990) canvassed, via mail, 25 000 Canadians of whom approximately 80% had MS. Using the Perceived Deficits Questionnaire, subjects were asked to rate their cognitive performance on four indices: attention, retrospective memory, prospective memory and planning/organizational skills. Five per cent (n=1180) of the sample responded, of whom 38% considered themselves cognitively impaired in at least one area. This figure approximates those from two large community-based neuropsychological studies (Rao et al., 1991a; McIntosh-Michaelis et al., 1991)(see section on prevalence of cognitive impairment). Whether the two assessment procedures are identifying the same group of patients must, however, be open to doubt, given the documented evidence of metamemory problems in MS patients. Sullivan et al.'s study was unable to provide the answer because objective assessment procedures were not undertaken. McIntosh-Michaelis et al. (1991), on the other hand, demonstrated convincingly that MS patients tended to substantially overestimate their perceptions of memory impairment and difficulties with attention.

In contrast to these findings, Kujala et al. (1996) found that MS patients with early cognitive decline were able to accurately appraise their memory deficits, which may indicate that metamemory is, in part, related to the overall severity of cognitive deficits.

Concept formation and abstract reasoning

Prompted by an observation of Canter (1951) that, in MS, 'the most striking psychological loss is inability to analyse and synthesize abstract problems' researchers have set about providing further empirical proof. The earliest attempt was by Parsons et al. (1957) who used the Grassi Block Substitution

Test (GBST), which requires the subject to shift construct several times at both a simple and complex level during a series of duplications of block designs.

Contrasting the performance of 17 MS patients (with the unusual gender distribution of 14 males and 3 females; the study took place in a V.A. Hospital) with 14 males and 3 female patients without CNS involvement recruited from the general medical wards, all subjects initially completed the verbal subscale of the Wechsler–Bellevue Intelligence Scale and four of the performance subscales, excluding Block Design test. Following this, all subjects were given the GBST in which they had to copy five designs of varying difficulty by utilizing four coloured blocks. Cognizant of potential motor difficulties in the MS group, subjects were allowed 5 minutes, as opposed to the usual 3 minutes, to complete each step. Analysing the results revealed significant deficits in the MS group, although taking into account the broad standard deviations, there was a degree of overlap in performance between the two groups. These differences could not be ascribed to IQ deficits in the MS patients, as the two groups were evenly matched for verbal scores. Although the MS patients had lower performance IQs, the authors controlled for this by taking a subgroup of nine MS patients whose performance IQs matched those of the controls. Once again, the MS patients demonstrated significantly more deficits. In keeping with results from other cognitive paradigms, there was a subgroup of MS patients whose performances showed no impairment.

Since then, a number of studies have replicated this finding using a different task of abstracting ability, namely the Wisconsin Card Sort Test (WCST), with Berg's (1948) original test giving way to a revised and expanded methodology (Heaton, 1981). Given the frequency with which this test has been used in MS research, a description of the methodology appears warranted. A subject is given a pack of 128 cards, which contain four symbols (star, cross, triangle and circle) in four colours (red, blue, green, yellow). Four stimulus cards are placed before the subject in the following left to right order: one red triangle, two green stars, three yellow crosses, four blue circles. The subject is then instructed to match each consecutive card from the deck with one of the four stimulus cards, in whichever way he thinks they match. The subject is only told whether he is right or wrong, and the correct sorting principle is never divulged. Once a certain number of correct responses are made to the initial sorting principle, the sorting principle is changed, e.g. from colour to form. This occurs without warning and the subject has only the examiner's responses to alert him to the change. The tests proceeds in similar fashion through a number of shifts in set, namely form, colour and number. The test provides scores on such indices as the number of categories completed, the total number of errors made and the number of perseverative errors made, to name three of the most sensitive markers of deficits in conceptual reasoning.

The WCST has proved effective in differentiating MS patients from healthy controls (Heaton et al., 1985, Beatty et al., 1989b; Rao et al., 1991a; Mendozzi et al., 1993) and disabled patients without brain involvement (Rao et al., 1987; Ron et al., 1991). The evidence that patients with chronic–progressive disease are more impaired than those with a relapsing–remitting course is equivocal, with Rao et al. (1987), but not Heaton et al. (1985) reporting intergroup differences, although the latter noted a trend for more errors in the chronic–progressive group.

There is confirmatory evidence from other similar neuropsychological tests that MS patients have difficulty problem solving, with a tendency to perseverate in their responses. This has been demonstrated with the Raven's Progressive Matrices (Rao et al., 1991a) and the Category Test (Peyser et al., 1980; Heaton et al., 1985; Rao et al., 1991a). All these tests are, however, measures of non-verbal abstracting ability prompting Beatty et al. (1995) to investigate whether MS patients confront similar difficulties with verbal abstraction. Their tests included two non-verbal measures, i.e. the WCST and a shortened version of the California Card Sort Test (CCST) and one verbal measure of abstracting ability, i.e. the Shipley Institute of Living Scale (SILS). The SILS measures both concept formation and abstracting ability, while taking into account overall verbal (vocabulary) performance. In relation to healthy controls, MS patient were impaired across all three measures. Their deficits on the SILS went beyond problems with vocabulary and illustrated that MS patients solve verbal abstraction problems more slowly and less accurately than controls.

Beatty and Monson (1996) have commented on a potential shortcoming of the WCST, which is the close correlation between the number of concepts attained and the number of perseverative responses made. The CCST, on the other hand, allows problem solving to be broken down into constituent processes that are, in theory, more independent. The examination therefore, provides separate assessments of concept generation, concept identification, and concept execution, in addition to various measures of perseveration. Comparing the performances of MS patients on the WCST and the CCST has led Beatty and Monson (1996) to conclude that the primary difficulty faced by MS patients when it comes to problem solving is difficulty with identifying concepts, rather than perseveration.

'Frontal lobe' tasks

While there is a consensus that MS patients as a group experience difficulties with abstraction and shifting set, what this means in terms of regional cerebral abnormalities is less clear. This is particularly relevant with respect to the WSCT, the most widely used test of abstraction in MS patients. Performance on the WCST has been thought to be dependent on the functional integrity of the dorsolateral prefrontal cortex (DLPFC), although there are dissenting voices (Andersen et al., 1991). Weinberger et al. (1986) using Positron Emission Tomography (PET) demonstrated that the inability of schizophrenic patients to match the performance of healthy controls on the WCST was associated with hypoperfusion of the DLPFC during task activation. Since then, however, it has become apparent that discrete anatomical circuits link areas of the prefrontal cortex (i.e. DLPFC, orbitofrontal cortex and anterior cingulate) with the basal ganglia and thalamus, before the circuit loops back to prefrontal areas (Cummings, 1993). The functional implications of these findings are that lesions remote from the prefrontal cortex may produce behavioural syndromes and cognitive difficulties (such as impairment on the WCST) that are identical to those associated with lesions localized to prefrontal areas. Empirical evidence that difficulties with abstract thinking (and perseverative responses) are also indicative of generalized cerebral dysfunction comes from Mendozzi et al. (1993). Although they noted that approximately a third of MS patients were impaired on the WCST relative to a healthy control group, performance on the WCST could not predict performance on other aspects of frontal lobe function as assessed by Luria–Nebraska Neuropsychological Battery. A critique of their finding is that it contains an unproven a priori assumption, namely that the LNNB frontal scale is a more valid measure of frontal function.

An analogous position exists with measures of verbal fluency. The Controlled Oral Word Association Test (COWAT) (Benton and Hamsher, 1976) has been widely used in MS patients. It consists of three-word naming trials, and the letters most frequently used are F, A and S. Subject are asked to generate as many words as they can think of beginning with the chosen letter, excluding proper nouns, numbers and the same word with a different suffix. A minute is allowed for each letter and the total score represents the summation of all words generated in the 3–minute period. Published normative data are available for comparisons. The test has been regarded as a sensitive indicator of brain dysfunction, in particular dominant frontal lobe pathology (Miceli et al., 1981), although Benton (1968) found that bilateral frontal lesions produced the most impaired scores. Verbal fluency is adversely affected in MS patients (Caine et al., 1986; Beatty et al., 1989a; Rao et al., 1991a), and the sensitivity of tests such as the COWAT in detecting cognitive impairment in MS has led to its inclusion in brief cognitive screening procedures for MS (Rao et al., 1991a; Basso et al., 1996).

However, like many good cognitive screening instruments, the COWAT taps more than a single aspect of cognition and is therefore likely to defy easy localization. Consequently, it may also be used as a cognitive screening test for the cortical dementias (Hart et al., 1988). Crawford et al. (1992) have demonstrated that scores correlate significantly with premorbid IQ as measured by a reading test such as the NART. This observation has generated data that allows the neuropsychiatrist to predict FAS scores on the basis of estimates of premorbid IQ (Crawford et al., 1992). Discrepancies between actual and predicted scores are thus another useful measure of general decline in intellect.

Reviewing data from such 'frontal' tests as the WCST and COWAT, one can only concur with Beatty (1993) that at present there is an inability to localize brain regions responsible for particular cognitive functions with any degree of anatomical precision.

Attention and information processing speed

Slowness of thinking, observed Charcot, was one of the hallmarks of mentation in MS patients. A century later, Cummings (1986) reiterated the significance of the symptom and went on to suggest it was one of the defining features of a broad category of dementing illnesses that were primarily subcortical in origin. Speed of information processing has been assessed in MS patients with a number of different tests of which the symbol-digit modality test (SDMT) is one of the most widely used. The test requires subjects to substitute numbers for symbols and responses are timed. Instead of writing their answers, subjects may respond orally, thereby removing the motor component to testing. Many studies have reported deficits in MS patients (Caine et al., 1986; Franklin et al., 1988; Feinstein et al., 1992a, 1993), and the test is recommended as a sensitive screening procedure for cognitive deficits (Beatty and Goodkin, 1990).

Another measure of cognitive speed is provided by the Paced Auditory Serial Addition Task (PASAT)(Gronwall and Wrightson, 1974). Initially devised as a means of assessing cognitive difficulties following traumatic brain injury, it has since been applied to other neurological disorders. In this test, subjects are presented aurally with a series of digits from 1 to 9 and instructed to add each new digit to the one that preceded it. The speed at which the digits are presented can be controlled and has generally varied from 1.2 seconds to 4 seconds. It is at the quicker rate that deficits become more readily apparent. Abnormalities on the PASAT in MS patients have been reported in numerous studies (Litvan et al., 1988a; Rao et al., 1991a; Feinstein et al., 1992a, 1993). In addition, a visual adaptation of the PASAT, whereby the numbers are presented on a computer monitor, has been developed and has replicated the auditory findings (Feinstein et al., 1992a).

In a study that specifically addressed the question of speed of information processing MS, Litvan et al. (1988a) reported mixed results. They found that patients were impaired compared to healthy controls on the PASAT when digits were presented at rapid (1.2 and 1.6 seconds), but not at slower rates (2.0 and 2.4 seconds). However, there were no significant differences between the two groups on another measure of cognitive speed, namely the Reed–Sternberg paradigm, which measures the rate at which subjects scan their immediate memory as part of digit recall. As a rule, the more digits subjects are required to remember, the longer it takes to scan their memory when presented with a probe digit. For younger subjects there is a 30 ms increase in reaction time for every additional digit added to the list they have to scan. An advantage to this particular test is that performance is independent of arithmetic or perceptual abilities. Why MS subjects should have been impaired on one, but not the other test of information processing speed was put down to the greater cognitive complexity of a task such as the PASAT, which assesses not only cognitive speed, but also arithmetic skills and the ability to retrieve information from short-term memory. It is also potentially influenced by perceptual abnormalities, be they auditory or visual.

This result has been disputed by two studies using the Reed–Sternberg paradigm, that both demonstrated significantly slowed scanning of working memory in MS patients (Rao et al., 1989a, 1991a). This makes the failure of the Litvan et al. (1988a) study perplexing. Type 11 error is unlikely, given their significant PASAT result. Similarly, the lesser degree of physical disability in their sample relative to the other studies is not a convincing argument, given the weak association between cognitive impairment and physical disability in MS in general.

An indirect measure of assessing information processing speed is via the use of simple (SRT) and choice (CRT) reaction time tests. In the former, subjects have only to respond to a stimulus, for example the appearance of a symbol on a computer monitor, by pressing a button. The responses are timed and the test is thus a measure of basic psychomotor speed. In the choice reaction time test, subjects are presented with a choice of responses, only one of which is correct. An element of problem solving is therefore introduced. By subtracting the SRT from the CRT, a measure of pure cognitive speed can be obtained. MS patients perform more slowly than controls on measures of psychomotor speed (Elsass and Zeeberg, 1983; Jennekens-Schinkel et al., 1988a). In keeping with these data, a significant association has also been noted between the degree of physical disability and slowed reaction times (Jennekens-Schinkel et al., 1988a).

However, when the complexity of the task was increased, i.e. the addition of a choice reaction component, further slowing in MS patients in relation to a control group was not reported (Jennekens-Schinkel et al., 1988b). Similarly, A. Feinstein et al. (unpublished data) did not find a significant difference between MS patients and an individually matched healthy control group on CRT–SRT times. Although some individual differences were obscured by the overall group data, problems with this approach are that it lacks the sensitivity of tests such as the PASAT and Reed–Sternberg paradigm, while also introducing the potential confounder of fatigue. The latter is endorsed by over 80% of MS patients (Krupp et al., 1988) and may adversely affect 'vigilance', defined as the ability to attend to a stimulus over time. Evidence of the role played by fatigue on attentional processes in MS comes from a study by Kujala et al. (1995). The performance of three groups, mildly cognitively impaired MS, cognitively intact MS and healthy controls, were compared on various measures of attention, vigilance and information processing speed (PASAT, Stroop colour-word test, auditory As and auditory trails A). The findings illustrated a two-way split, in that cognitively intact MS patients demonstrated signs of motor and fatigue-related slowness, whereas the mildly cognitively impaired group demonstrated more prominent features of cognitive slowness.

A second study by Kujala et al. (1994) investigated information processing speed by dividing it into three separate stages. The first division refers to automatic processing of information and does not require conscious effort. An example given is the recognition of numbers presented in the centre of the visual field. The second stage is one of controlled processing and demands not only attention, but also working memory. An example is conscious decision making, which can be tested with choice reaction time tasks. The third component is motor programming, which refers to the time a subject needs to prepare a motor programme before executing a task. This too is assumed to be automatic. The authors investigated these three aspects in two matched MS samples, one deemed cognitively intact and the other mildly impaired. Not surprisingly, the latter performed more poorly at every stage of processing information, but of additional note was that MS subjects thought to be cognitively preserved also showed mild slowing in automatic processing. This finding does not contradict the assertions of Beatty et al. (1990a) and Grafman et al. (1991) that automatic processes such as priming and condioned responses, all part of implicit memory, are intact, for these measure essentially separate aspects of automatic processing. What the study does, however, suggest is that slowing of information processing may be due, in part, to the slowness of the visual input system, i.e. delayed conduction in the optic nerves in the absence of discernable cerebral involvement may still produce subtle deficits.

The relationship of cognition to other aspects of MS

Depression

Depression masquerading as dementia is a frequently encountered problem in a neuropsychiatric setting. Depression often accompanies cognitive dysfunction (Caine, 1981) and in some cases may be the harbinger of intellectual difficulties that will only become apparent in time. There are, however, some clues from history and mental state examination that point to a primary mood change and these include a family history of affective disorder and a preserved ability to learn new information. Neuropsychological testing may further help in diagnostic clarification. A three-way comparison of memory testing in brain-damaged, depressed and healthy controls has demonstrated clear performance differences in the brain damaged patients and has shown that depression is unlikely to significantly compromise performance (Coughlan and Hollows, 1984). Similar conclusions apply to multiple sclerosis patients. Although MS patients display a high lifetime prevalence rate of clinically significant depression (see Chapter 2), the mood change is unlikely to impinge on memory. This conclusion holds irrespective of whether depression is diagnosed via the preferred method of direct clinical interview (Lyon-Caen et al., 1986; Möller et al., 1994), or according to a less valid approach, namely scores on self-report rating scales (Beatty et al. 1988; Fischer, 1988; Rao et al., 1991a).

Schiffer and Caine (1991) investigated whether clinically significant depression (i.e. major depression) could affect cognitive performance, by testing MS patients when they were depressed and, on average, 7 months later when their mood state had resolved. No significant differences were found. A trend for verbal memory to improve was possibly due to the effects of practice, and the authors concluded that mood change in MS exerted little effect on cognition.

Medication

To what extent psychotropic medication may influence cognitive performance is an important consideration and one of practical importance, given the high psychiatric morbidity associated with MS. In a study of 92 community-based MS patients one-third were found to be taking tranquillizers, 7% either antidepressants or neuroleptics and 2% morphine. Twenty one per cent used medication that was non-sedative and only a third of patients were medication free (Stenager et al., 1994). However, when tested with an array of neuropsychological tests, including the Symbol Digit Modality Test as a measure of information processing speed, no association was found between cognitive performance and the use of sedative medication. Lack of a specific association between medication effects and cognitive performance has also been reported by Rao et al. (1991a).

Physical disability

The study of the relationship between cognitive dysfunction and physical disability has yielded contradictory findings (Heaton et al., 1985; Rao et al., 1991a). In a study designed specifically to address this relationship, Marsh (1980) found that disability as measured by the Kurtzke Disability Scale (KDS)(Kurtzke 1970) correlated only with duration of illness, but not with either verbal, performance or full scale IQ on the WAIS. She did, however, note that scores on performance subtests with a large motor component were lower than the verbal subsets. A failure to find any association between KDS (Kurtzke, 1970) scores and cognitive function has also been reported by others (Peyser et al., 1980; Rao et al., 1985; Lyon-Caen et al., 1986). Alternative procedures for assessing physical disability such as the Activities of Daily Living Test (Howarth and Hollings, 1979) have given similar results (Ron et al., 1991).

There are, however, exceptions to the above (Huber et al., 1987; Stenager et al., 1989), while indirect support has also come from Beatty and Gange (1979), who used five measures of motor impairment and found a correlation with memory deficits. An epidemiological study investigating the frequency, patterns and predictors of cognitive dysfunction (Rao et al., 1991a), noted a weak, but significant, correlation with disability.

Failure to find an association may be an artefact of research methodology that relies on a biased rating assessment procedure. Thus, while cognitive deficits are attributable to plaques in the cerebral hemisphere white matter, physical disability as measured by the scales such as the KDS (Kurtzke, 1970) or EDSS (Kurtzke, 1983) predominantly reflects the presence of lesions in the spinal cord, posterior fossa and cerebellum, causing mainly motor effects (see Chapter 1 for a critique of the Kurtzke scales). A further problem in interpreting these data is that physical disability is often linked to variables such as age, exacerbation, disease duration and disease course. Thus, more disabled patients have tended to be older with disease of longer duration and a chronic–progressive course. To separate these potentially confounding effects, Beatty et al. (1990b) undertook a longitudinal study, whereby disease type was only assigned after a 2-year period, during which patients underwent neurological examination every 6 months. Using multiple regression techniques, they failed to find any demographic or clinical predictors of cognitive performance.

Duration of illness

The majority of studies have failed to find an association between disease duration and cognitive dysfunction (Ivnik, 1978; Rao et al., 1984, 1985, 1991a). Marsh (1980), although finding a link between disease duration and disability, found that neither correlated with cognition. The reason for this can be traced to the fact that patients with illnesses of similar durations may differ greatly with respect to disease activity, ranging from quiescent ('benign') to rapidly progressive. Controlling for confounding effects such as age and disease course (Beatty et al., 1990b) also failed to demonstrate such a relationship.

There are, however, a minority of studies that have reported different results. Ron et al. (1991) found a positive association with a modest correlation coefficient (r=0.30), albeit significant at a 1% level while Grant et al. (1984) showed that disturbances in short-term memory, learning and recall of verbal and non-verbal information were associated with the number of years of 'active disease'. They defined this concept as the 'number of years in which the patient reported at least one week's duration of symptoms', which is open to criticism as MRI studies have shown that clinical relapses do not often mirror the development of new brain lesions, the latter occurring seven times more often (Thompson et al., 1992).

Disease course

Initial evidence suggested that cognitive deficits were more marked in patients with chronic–progressive as opposed to relapsing–remitting, MS. Heaton et al. (1985) studied 100 patients with either relapsing–remitting (RR)(N=57) or chronic–progressive (CP) MS, who were consecutive admissions to a neurological ward and a similar number of healthy controls. Patients were clinically stable at the time of testing. Both the CP and RR groups were more cognitively impaired than the group of healthy controls, and the CP patients were, in turn, more cognitively impaired than RR patients on most measures. These differences were not related to greater sensory or motor impairment in the CP group and persisted when the duration of disease (longer in the CP group) was controlled for.

This result was confirmed by Rao et al. (1987), who compared the performances of RR and CP patients and a control group of back pain sufferers using the Wisconsin Card Sort Test. Whilst no differences were apparent between the RR group and control subjects, CP patients differed from both in terms of the number of perseverative errors and fewer categories achieved. A stepwise regression analysis suggested that these differences were independent of physical disability or disease duration.

Indirect evidence supporting disease course, as an important predictor of cognitive dysfunction, has also come from studies confined to one of the subgroups. Thus, in a study of RR patients, Anzola et al. (1990) reported a mild overall cognitive impairment, while Beatty et al. (1989a) observed that cognitive deficits in their RR patients were less severe than those previously documented in subjects with a CP course. Studies limited to CP patients have reported that three-quarters were impaired on tests of information processing speed (Beatty et al., 1988) and that memory was significantly compromised in over half (Rao et al., 1984).

However, all these findings linking cognition to a CP disease course were reported prior to longitudinal studies being undertaken. Follow-up studies have revealed a different picture (Jennekens-Schinkel et al., 1990), namely that the crucial variable in determining cognitive change is not disease course, but lesion load in the brain (Feinstein et al., 1992b, 1993; Hohol et al., 1997). While a CP course may be frequently associated with more extensive brain plaques, this is not invariably so. In addition, if the lesion burden falls predominantly within the spinal cord, disease course becomes less relevant with respect to cognition. Longitudinal studies have also called into question assumptions that the course of MS runs true once established. In a 1- to 5-year follow-up study (mean 2.6 years) of 254 patients with definite MS, Goodkin et al. (1989) found that approximately a third of CP patients became stable, while slightly less (20%) RR patients deteriorated to a CP course. It should be noted, however, that no patients reverted from a CP to a RR course. Nevertheless, the data further question whether a clear-cut relationship between disease course and cognitive impairment exists. Beatty et al. (1990b), using the same patient data-base reported by Goodkin and colleagues, assigned disease course to patients only after a minimum 2 years observation. Forty-two and 43 patients with RR and CP MS, respectively, were then selected to undergo psychometric assessment. Using multiple regression techniques, disease course was an excellent predictor of physical disability (accounting for greater than 50% of the variance), but no variable was found to be a significant predictor of cognitive dysfunction.

Summary

- The prevalence of cognitive dysfunction in a representative, community-based sample of MS patients is approximately 40%.
- Decline in intellect (IQ) does occur, but is mainly related to measures on the performance subscale.
- Memory function has been well studied and reveals that short-term deficits, although present, are less marked than those affecting long-term memory. Verbal and non-verbal memory are adversely affected and the mechanism involves failure both at the acquisition and retrieval stages. Deficits are, however, more apparent on tests of recall than recognition. Metamemory too is impaired, but implicit memory appears largely spared.
- Hallmarks of cognitive dysfunction are a reduced speed of information processing and impaired attention.
- Well-described deficits are present on tests of executive function, where the predominant problem may be generating concepts as opposed to perseverative responses.

- Cognitive dysfunction is not closely associated with physical disability, disease duration or disease course.
- Cognitive dysfunction cannot be accounted for by depression nor by the presence of psychotropic medication.

References

Albert ML, Feldman RG, Willis AL. (1974) The 'subcortical dementia' of progressive supranuclear palsy. *Journal of Neurology, Neurosurgery and Psychiatry*, **37**, 121–30.

Anzola GP, Bevilacqua L, Cappa SF et al. (1990) Neuropsychological assessment in patients with relapsing–remitting multiple sclerosis and mild functional impairment: correlation with magnetic resonance imaging. *Journal of Neurology, Neurosurgery and Psychiatry*, **53**, 142–5.

Anderson SW, Damasio H, Jones RD, Tranel D. (1991) Wisconsin Card Sorting Test performance as a measure of frontal lobe damage. *Journal of Clinical and Experimental Neuropsychology*, **13**, 909–22.

Baddeley A. (1986) *Working Memory*. New York: Oxford University Press.

Basso MR, Beason-Hazen S, Lynn J, Rammohan K, Bornstein RA. (1996) Screening for cognitive dysfunction in multiple sclerosis. *Archives of Neurology*, **53**, 980–4.

Beatty WW (1993) Memory and 'frontal lobe' dysfunction in multiple sclerosis. *Journal of Neurological Sciences*, **115** (Suppl.), 38–41.

Beatty PA, Gange JJ. (1979) Neuropsychological aspects of multiple sclerosis. *Journal of Nervous and Mental Disease*, **164**, 42–50.

Beatty WW, Goodkin DE. (1990) Screening for cognitive impairment in multiple sclerosis. An evaluation of the mini-mental state examination. *Archives of Neurology*, **47**, 297–301.

Beatty WW, Monson N. (1990) Semantic priming in multiple sclerosis. Bulletin of the *Psychonomic Society*, **28**, 397–400.

Beatty WW, Monson N.(1991) Metamemory in multiple sclerosis. *Journal of Clinical and Experimental Neuropsychology*, **13**, 309–27.

Beatty WW, Monson N. (1996) Problem solving by patients with multiple sclerosis: Comparison of performance on the Wisconsin and California card sorting tests. *Journal of the International Neuropsychological Society*, **2**, 134–40.

Beatty WW, Goodkin DE, Monson N, Beatty PA. (1990a) Implicit learning in patients with chronic–progressive multiple sclerosis. *International Journal of Clinical Neuropsychology*, **12**, 153–62.

Beatty WW, Goodkin DE, Monson N, Beatty PA. (1989a) Cognitive disturbance in patients with relapsing–remitting multiple sclerosis. *Archives of Neurology*, **46**, 1113–19.

Beatty WW, Goodkin DE, Beatty PA, Monson N. (1989b) Frontal lobe dysfunction and memory impairment in patients with chronic–progressive multiple sclerosis. *Brain and Cognition*, **11**, 73–86.

Beatty WW, Goodkin DE, Monson N, Beatty PA, Hertsgaard D. (1988) Anterograde and retrograde amnesia in patients with chronic–progressive multiple sclerosis. *Archives of Neurology*, **45**, 611–19.

Beatty WW, Hames KA, Blanco CR, Paul RH, Wilbanks SL (1995) Verbal abstraction deficit in multiple sclerosis. *Neuropsychology*, **9**, 198–205.

Beatty WW, Wilbanks SL, Bianco CR, Hames KA, Tivis R, Paul RH. (1996) Memory disturbance in multiple sclerosis: reconsideration of patterns of performance on the selective reminding test. *Journal of Clinical and Experimental Neuropsychology*, **18**, 56–62.

Beatty WW, Goodkin DE, Hertsgaard D, Monson N. (1990b) Clinical and demographic predictors of cognitive performance in MS. Do diagnostic type, disease duration and disability matter? *Archives of Neurology*, **47**, 305–8.

Benton AL. (1968) Differential behavioural effects of frontal lobe disease. *Neuropsychologia*, **6**, 53–60.

Benton AL, Hamsher KdeS. (1976) *Multilingual Aphasia Examination*. Iowa City, IA: University of Iowa Press.

Berg EAA. (1948) A simple objective test for measuring flexibility in thinking. *Journal of General Psychology*, **39**, 15–22.

Caine ED (1981) Pseudodementia: current concepts and future directions. *Archives of General Psychiatry*, **38**, 1359–64.

Caine ED, Bamford KA, Schiffer RB, Shoulson I, Levy S. (1986) A controlled neuropsychological comparison of Huntington's disease and multiple sclerosis. *Archives of Neurology*, **43**, 249–54.

Canter AH (1951) Direct and indirect measures of psychological deficit in multiple sclerosis. Part 1. *The Journal of General Psychology*, **44**, 3–25.

Carroll M, Gates R, Roldan F. (1984) Memory impairment in multiple sclerosis. *Neuropsychologia*, **22**, 297–302.

Charcot J-M. (1877) *Lectures on the Diseases of the Nervous System delivered at La Salpetriere*. pp. 194–5. London: New Sydenham Society.

Cottrell SS, Wilson SAK (1926) The affective symptomatology of disseminated multiple sclerosis. *Journal of Neurological Psychopathology*, **7**, 1–30.

Coughlan AK, Hollows SE. (1984) Use of memory tests in differentiating organic disorder from depression. *British Journal of Psychiatry*, **145**, 164–7.

Crawford JR, Moore JW, Cameron IM. (1992) Verbal fluency: a NART-based equation for the estimation of premorbid performance. *British Journal of Clinical Psychology*, **31**, 327–9.

Cummings JL. (1986) Subcortical dementia. Neuropsychology, neuropsychiatry, and pathophysiology. *British Journal of Psychiatry*, **149**, 682–97.

Cummings JL (1993) Frontal subcortical circuits and human behaviour. *Archives of Neurology*, **50**, 873–80.

D'Esposito M, Onishi K, Thompson H, Robinson K, Armstrong C, Grossman M. (1996) Working memory impairments in multiple sclerosis: evidence from a dual-task paradigm. *Neuropsychology*, **10**, 51–6.

DeLucca J, Barbieri-Berger S, Johnson SK. (1994) The nature of memory impairment in multiple sclerosis: acquisition versus retrieval. *Journal of Clinical and Experimental Neuropsychology*, **16**, 183–9.

Elsass P, Zeeberg I. (1983) Reaction time deficit in multiple sclerosis. *Acta Neurologica Scandinavica*, **68**, 257–61.

Feinstein A, Feinstein KJ, Gray T, O'Connor P. (1997) Neurobehavioural correlates of pathological crying and laughing in multiple sclerosis. *Archives of Neurology*, **54**,

1116–21.

Feinstein A, Kartsounis L, Miller D, Youl B, Ron M. (1992b) Clinically isolated lesions of the type seen in multiple sclerosis followed up: a cognitive, psychiatric and MRI study. *Journal of Neurology, Neurosurgery and Psychiatry*, **55**, 869–76.

Feinstein A, Ron M, Thompson A. (1993) A serial study of psychometric and magnetic resonance imaging changes in multiple sclerosis. *Brain*, **116**, 569–602.

Feinstein A, Youl B, Ron M. (1992a) Acute optic neuritis. A cognitive and magnetic resonance imaging study. *Brain*, **115**, 1403–15.

Fink SL, Houser HB. (1966) An investigation of physical and intellectual changes in multiple sclerosis. *Archives of Physical Medicine and Rehabilitation*, **47**, 56–61.

Fischer J. (1988) Using the Wechsler Memory Scale – Revised to detect and characterize memory deficits in multiple sclerosis. *Clinical Neuropsychology*, **2**, 149–72.

Fischer J, Kawczak K, Daughtry MM, Schwetz KM, Rudick RA, Goodkin DE. (1992). Unmasking subtypes of verbal memory impairment in multiple sclerosis. *Journal of Clinical and Experimental Neuropsychology*, **14**, 32.

Folstein MF, Folstein SE, McHugh PR. (1975) 'Mini-Mental State': a practical method for grading the cognitive state of patients for the clinician. *Journal of Psychiatric Research*, **12**, 189–98.

Franklin GM, Heaton RK, Nelson LM, Filley CM, Seibert C. (1988) Correlation of neuropsychological and MRI findings in chronic–progressive multiple sclerosis. *Neurology*, **38**, 1826–9.

Goldstein G, Shelly (1974) Neuropsychological diagnosis of multiple sclerosis in a neuropsychiatric setting. *Journal of Nervous and Mental Disease*, **158**, 280–90.

Goldstein FC, McKendall RR, Haut MC. (1992) Gist recall in multiple sclerosis. *Archives of Neurology*, **49**, 1060–4.

Goodkin DE, Hertsgaard D, Rudick RA. (1989) Exacerbation rates and adherence to disease type in a prospectively followed-up population with multiple sclerosis. *Archives of Neurology*, **46**, 1107–12.

Grafman J. Rao S, Bernardin L, Leo GJ. (1991) Automatic memory processes in patients with multiple sclerosis. *Archives of Neurology*, **48**, 1072–5.

Grafman J, Rao SM, Litvan I. (1990) Disorders of memory. in *Neurobehavioural Aspects of Multiple Sclerosis*, ed. S Rao. New York: Oxford University Press.

Grant I, McDonald WI, Trimble MR, Smith E, Reed R. (1984) Deficient learning and memory in early and middle phases of multiple sclerosis. *Journal of Neurology, Neurosurgery and Psychiatry*, **47**, 25–55.

Gronwall DMA, Wrightson P. (1974) Delayed recovery of intellectual function after minor head injury. *Lancet*, **ii**, 605–9.

Hart S, Smith CM, Swash M. (1988) Word fluency in patients with early dementia of Alzheimer type. *British Journal of Clinical Psychology*, **28**, 115–24.

Heaton RK (1981) Wisconsin Card Sorting Test Manual. Odessa, FL: *Psychological Assessment Resources*.

Heaton RK, Nelson LM, Thompson DS, Burk JS, Franklin GM. (1985) Neuropsychological findings in relapsing–remitting and chronic–progressive multiple sclerosis. *Journal of Consulting and Clinical Psychology*, **53**, 103–10.

Hodges JR. (1994) *Cognitive Assessment for Clinicians*. Oxford: Oxford University Press.

Hohol MJ, Guttmann CRG, Orav GA et al. (1997) Serial neuropsychological assessment and magnetic resonance imaging analysis in multiple sclerosis. *Archives of Neurology*, **54**, 1018–25.

Howarth RJ, Hollings EM. (1979) Are hospital assessments of daily living activities valid? *International Rehabilitation Medicine*, **1**, 59–62.

Huber SJ, Paulsen GW, Suttleworth EC et al. (1987) Magnetic resonance imaging correlates of dementia in multiple sclerosis. *Archives of Neurology*, **44**, 732–6.

Ivnik RJ. (1978) Neuropsychological test performance as a function of the duration of MS related symptomatology. *The Journal of Clinical Psychiatry*, **39**, 304–12.

Jambor KL. (1969) Cognitive functioning in multiple sclerosis. *British Journal of Psychiatry*, **115**, 765–75.

Jennekens-Schinkel A, Laboyrie PM, Lanser JBK, van der Velde EA. (1990) Cognition in patients with multiple sclerosis after 4 years. *Journal of the Neurological Sciences*, **99**, 229–47.

Jennekens-Schinkel A, Sanders EACM, Lanser JBK, van der Velde EA. (1988a) Reaction time in ambulant multiple sclerosis patients. Part 1. Influence of prolonged cognitive effort. *Journal of the Neurological Sciences*, **85**, 173–86.

Jennekens-Schinkel A, Sanders EACM, Lanser JBK, van der Velde EA. (1988b) Reaction time in ambulant multiple sclerosis patients. Part II. Influence of task complexity. *Journal of the Neurological Sciences*, **85**, 187–96.

Kahana EK, Leibowitz U, Alter M (1971) Cerebral multiple sclerosis. *Neurology*, **21**, 1179–85.

Krupp LB, Alvarez LA, LaRocca N, Scheinberg LC. (1988) Fatigue in multiple sclerosis. *Archives of Neurology*, **45**, 435–7.

Kurtzke JF. (1970) Neurologic impairment in multiple sclerosis and the Disability Status Score. *Acta Neurologica Scandinavica*, **46**, 493–512.

Kurtzke JF (1983) Rating neurologic impairment in multiple sclerosis: an expanded disability scale. *Neurology*, **33**, 1444–52.

Kujala P, Portin R, Revonsuo A, Ruutiainen J. (1994) Automatic and controlled information processing in multiple sclerosis. *Brain*, **117**, 1115–26.

Kujala P, Portin R, Revonsuo A, Ruutiainen J. (1995) Attention related performance in two cognitively different subgroups of patients with multiple sclerosis. *Journal of Neurology, Neurosurgery and Psychiatry*, **59**, 77–82.

Kujala P, Portin R, Ruutiainen J. (1996) Memory deficits and early cognitve deterioration in MS. *Acta Neurologica Scandinavica*, **93**, 329–35.

Litvan I, Grafman J, Vendrell P, Martinez JM. (1988a) Slowed information processing speed in multiple sclerosis. *Archives of Neurology*, **45**, 281–5.

Litvan I, Grafman J, Vendrell P et al. (1988b) Multiple memory deficits in patients with multiple sclerosis. Exploring the working memory system. *Archives of Neurology*, **45**, 607–10.

Lyon-Caen O, Jouvent R, Hauser S et al. (1986) Cognitive function in recent onset demyelinating diseases. *Archives of Neurology*, **43**, 1138–41.

Marsh GG (1980) Disability and intellectual function in multiple sclerosis patients. *Journal of Nervous and Mental Disease*, **168**, 758–62.

Mendozzi L, Pugnetti L, Saccani M, Motta A. (1993) Frontal lobe dysfunction in multiple sclerosis as assessed by means of Lurian tasks: effects of age of onset. *Journal of Neurological Sciences*, **115** (Suppl), S42–S50.

McIntosh-Michaelis SA, Wilkinson SM, Diamond ID, McLellan DL, Martin JP and

Spackman AJ (1991) The prevalence of cognitive impairment in a community survey of multiple sclerosis. *British Journal of Clinical Psychology*, **30**, 333–48.

Miceli G, Caltagirone C, Gainotti G, Masullo C, Silveri MC. (1981) Neuropsychological correlates of localised cerebral lesions in non-aphasic brain damaged patients. *Journal of Clinical Neuropsychology*, **3**, 53–63.

Minden SL, Moes EJ, Orav J, Kaplan E, Reich P. (1990) Memory impairment in multiple sclerosis. *Journal of Clinical and Experimental Neuropsychology*, **12**, 566–86.

Möller A, Wiedemann G, Rohde U, Backmund H, Sonntag A. (1994) Correlates of cognitive impairment and depressive mood disorder in multiple sclerosis. *Acta Psychiatrica Scandinavica*, **89**, 117–21.

Nelson HE (1982) *National Adult Reading Test: Manual*. Windsor: NFER-Nelson.

Parsons OA, Stewart KD, Arenberg D. (1957) Impairment of abstracting ability in multiple sclerosis. *Journal of Nervous and Mental Disease*, **125**, 221–5.

Peyser JM, Edwards KR, Poser CM, Filskov SB. (1980) Cognitive function in patients with multiple sclerosis. *Archives of Neurology*, **37**, 577–9.

Peyser JM, Rao SM, LaRocca NG, Kaplan E. (1990) Guidelines for neuropsychological research in multiple sclerosis. *Archives of Neurology*, **47**, 94–7.

Rao SM (1986) Neuropsychology of multiple sclerosis. A critical review. *Journal of Clinical and Experimental Neuropsychology*, **8**, 503–42.

Rao SM, Glatt S, Hammeke TA et al. (1985) Chronic-progressive multiple sclerosis: relationship between cerebral ventricular size and neuropsychological impairment. *Archives of Neurology*, **42**, 678–82.

Rao SM, Hammeke TA, McQuillen MP, Khatri BO, Lloyd D. (1984) Memory disturbance in chronic–progressive multiple sclerosis. *Archives of Neurology*, **41**, 625–31.

Rao SM, Hammeke TA, Speech TJ (1987) Wisconsin Card Sort Test performance in relapsing–remitting and chronic–progressive multiple sclerosis. *Journal of Consulting and Clinical Psychology*, **55**, 263–5.

Rao SM, Leo GJ, Bernardin L, Unverzagt F. (1991a) Cognitive dysfunction in multiple sclerosis. 1. Frequency, patterns and prediction. *Neurology*, **41**, 685–91.

Rao SM, Leo GJ, Ellington L, Nauertz T, Bernardin L, Unverzagt F. (1991b) Cognitive dysfunction in multiple sclerosis. 11. Impact on employment and social functioning. *Neurology*, **41**, 692–6.

Rao SM, St. Aubin-Faubert P, Leo GJ. (1989a) Information processing speed in patients with multiple sclerosis. *Journal of Clinical and Experimental Neuropsychology*, **11**, 471–7.

Rao SM, Leo GJ, St. Aubin-Flaubert P. (1989b) On the nature of memory disturbance in multiple sclerosis. *Journal of Clinical and Experimental Neuropsychology*, **11**, 699–712,

Raven JC (1958) *Advanced Progressive Matrices Manual*. HK Lewis and Co: London.

Reitan RM, Reed JC, Dyken ML. (1971) Cognitive, psychomotor and motor correlates of multiple sclerosis. *Journal of Nervous and Mental Disease*, **153**, 218–24.

Ron MA, Callanan MM, Warrington EK. (1991) Cognitive abnormalities in multiple sclerosis. a psychometric and MRI study. *Psychological Medicine*, **21**, 59–68.

Schacter DL, Tulving E. (1994) *Memory Systems*. Cambridge, MA: The MIT Press.

Schiffer RB, Caine ED. (1991) The interaction between depressive affective disorder and neuropsychological test performance in multiple sclerosis. *The Journal of Neuropsychiatry and Clinical Neurosciences*, **3**, 28–32.

Shepherd D. (1979) Clinical features of multiple sclerosis in north east Scotland. *Acta Neurological Scandinavica*, **60**, 218–30.

Squire LR. (1987) *Memory and Brain*. New York: Oxford University Press.

Staples D, Lincoln NB. (1979) Intellectual impairment in multiple sclerosis and its relation to functional abilities. *Rheumatology and Rehabilitation*, **18**, 153–60.

Stenager E, Knudsen L, Jensen K. (1989) Correlation of Beck depression inventory score, Kurtzke disability status and cognitive functioning in multiple sclerosis. In *Current Problems in Neurology: 10. Mental Disorders and Cognitive Deficits in Multiple Sclerosis*, ed. K Jensen, L Knudsen, E Stenager, I Grant. London: John Libbey: pp. 147–52.

Stenager E, Knudsen L, Jensen K. (1994) Multiple sclerosis: methodological aspects of cognitive testing. *Acta Neurologica Belgica*, **94**, 53–6.

Sullivan MJL, Edgley K, Dehoux E. (1990) A survey of multiple sclerosis. Part 1: Perceived cognitive problems and compensatory strategy use. *Canadian Journal of Rehabilitation*, **4**, 99–105.

Taylor R. (1990) Relationships between cognitive test performance and everyday cognitive difficulties in multiple sclerosis. *British Journal of Clinical Psychology*, **29**, 251–2.

Thompson AJ, Miller D, Youl B et al. (1992) Serial gadolinium enhanced MRI in relapsing remitting multiple sclerosis of varying disease duration. *Neurology*, **42**, 60–3.

Thornton AE, Raz N. (1997) Memory impairment in multiple sclerosis. A quantitative review. *Neuropsychology*, B11, 357–66.

van den Burg W, van Zomeren AH, Minderhoud JM, Prange AJA, Meijer NSA (1987) Cognitive impairment in patients with multiple sclerosis and mild physical disability. *Archives of Neurology*, **44**, 494–501.

Wechsler D. (1955) *Wechsler Adult Intelligence Scale: Manual*. New York: Psychological Corporation.

Weinberger DR, Berman KF, Zec RF (1986) Physiologic dysfunction of the dorsolateral prefrontal cortex in schizophrenia. *Archives of General Psychiatry*, **43**, 114–24.

Wishart H, Sharpe D. (1997) Neuropsychological aspects of multiple sclerosis. *Journal of Clinical and Experimental Neuropsychology*, **19**, 810–24.

7

The natural history of cognitive change in multiple sclerosis

The initial cognitive studies in multiple sclerosis were concerned with establishing the prevalence and nature of the deficits. Once these objective had largely been attained, attention could be directed at other areas such as the pathogenesis, natural history, clinical significance, and treatment of cognitive difficulties. This chapter will review the findings relating to one of these respects, namely the natural history of cognitive decline in MS and attempt to answer the following questions. How early in the illness does cognitive dysfunction become apparent? How do these changes progress over the years or indeed, do they progress? With multiple sclerosis frequently running a relapsing–remitting course characterized by disease exacerbations and variable degrees of recovery, how do these changes affect cognition?

The onset of cognitive dysfunction

Canter (1951a,b) had shown that, within 4 years of developing MS, a general decline in intellect occurred. However, it was unclear whether cognitive decline coincided with the onset of neurological symptoms or at some point thereafter. In addition, the limited scope of Canter's psychometric battery and his failure to control for factors such as physical disability, disease course and exacerbations at the time of testing, introduced a note of caution when it came to data interpretation.

Clinically isolated lesions of the type seen in MS

In order to assess how early cognitive abnormalities become apparent, research has been directed at patients with clinically isolated lesions of the type seen in MS. These syndromes may present as optic neuritis, brainstem or spinal cord syndromes (see Chapter 1). Given that clinically isolated lesions (CIL) are frequently the harbinger of MS, the search for cognitive abnormalities in these patients may indicate how early in the disease process intellectual deficits begin. Callanan et al. (1989) studied a heterogenous group of 48 patients with CIL, composed almost equally of optic neuritis, brainstem and spinal cord presentations. Their mean duration of symptoms was 2.2 years and their performance on a number of cognitive indices were compared to a control group with physically disabling conditions sparing brain involvement (i.e. rheumatoid arthritis). The CIL group were found to have a greater decline in IQ and more deficits on tests of auditory attention than the control group. Of the CIL patients 81% had abnormalities on brain MRI, which correlated significantly with indices of cognitive dysfunction. The high number of patients with cerebral lesions is, however, unusual for a sample of patients with CIL and may relate to the mean 2-year duration of neurological symptoms prior to MR imaging.

The study replicated the results of earlier work by Lyon-Caen et al. (1986), who investigated the presence of cognitive and psychiatric abnormalities in nine patients with optic neuritis and 21 patients with definite or probable MS of less than 2 years' duration. Deficits were present in 60% of subjects, compared to a control group with neurological disorders such as headache, epilepsy and facial palsy. The optic neuritis patients were less cognitively impaired than the MS group, but both groups had deficits on a number of the subscales of the Wechsler Adult Intelligence Scale and the Wechsler Memory Scale.

While both the above studies pointed towards the development of cognitive dysfunction early in the disease process, the relatively long duration of symptoms prior to testing and, in the case of the Lyon Caen et al. study, the heterogenous nature of their sample, left unanswered the question whether cognitive changes were present at the outset of patients becoming neurologically symptomatic. This was addressed by Feinstein et al. (1992a) in a study of 42 patients with acute optic neuritis, whose mean duration of symptoms was 14 days. No subject had a duration of symptoms greater than 5 weeks, and subjects were excluded if the vision in the unaffected eye was less than 6/6. A battery of psychometric tests including an estimate of premorbid IQ, Purdue Pegboard Test Raven's matrices, Stroop Colour Word Test, Symbol-Digit Modalities Test (SDMT), The Paced Auditory Serial Addition Task (PASAT), The Paced Visual Serial Addition Task (PVSAT), and tests of Simple Reaction and Choice Reaction times were given to patients and a demographically matched group of healthy subjects. Subjects also underwent MRI of the brain and abnormalities noted in 55% of the sample.

A three-way cognitive comparison was undertaken between optic neuritis patients with and without brain lesions and the healthy control group. The results are displayed in Table 7.1 and illustrate that significant deficits in pegboard performance and auditory (PASAT) and visual (PVSAT) attention were present in the optic neuritis group, particularly if brain lesions were present. Tests such as the Stroop, SDMT, PASAT and PVSAT may be loosely grouped into the category 'tests of attention'. The fact that deficits were present in only some may be due to the greater complexity of those tasks. The failure of the optic neuritis group with brain lesions to perform adequately on the serial addition tasks may reflect, not only difficulties with attention, but

Table 7.1 Comparisons in cognition between healthy controls and optic neuritis patients with and without brain lesions on MRI

	Group 1: Controls (n=36) σ(sd) median (range)	Group 2: ON with normal MRI (n=19) σ(sd) median (range)	Group 3: ON with abnormal MRI (n=23) σ(sd) median (range)	One-way ANOVA/ Kruskal–Wallis	Sig.	1 vs 2	1 vs 3	2 vs 3
Pegboard test	41.8(4.4)	37.3(4.6)	37.7(4.6)	$F=9.0$	$P<0.0001$	+	+	.
Raven's matrices	11.4(3.0)	10.5(2.5)	10.1(2.6)	$F=1.9$	NS	.	.	.
Stroop test	22.4(4.8)	22.1(4.9)	25.1(7.0)	$F=2.1$	NS	.	.	.
SDMT	11.8(1.8)	12.0(1.0)	12.9(1.9)	$F=3.0$	$P<0.06$	.	.	.
PASAT (4 s)	2.0(0–8.0)	1.0(0–7.0)	3.0(0–14.0)	$x^2=7.3$	$P<0.03$	.	+	+
PASAT (2 s)	7.9(3.7)	8.1(4.4)	11.2(5.4)	$F=4.3$	$P<0.01$	.	+	.
PVSAT (4 s)	0.5(0–6.0)	0(0–5.0)	1.0(0–15.0)	$x^2=0.14$	NS	.	+	.
PVSAT (2 s)	4.8(3.4)	5.9(4.6)	7.8(4.6)	$F=3.7$	$P<0.03$	.	+	.

SDMT=symbol–digit substitution; PASAT=paced auditory serial addition task; PVSAT=paced visual serial addition task; s = time in seconds between the stimulus presentation; σ = mean; sd = standard deviation; Sig. = significance; the Stroop and SDMT scores are times (in seconds). Feinstein et al. (1992a). By permission of Oxford University Press.

also abnormalities in speed or efficiency of information processing, a function noted to be slowed in patients with a confirmed diagnosis of MS (see Chapter 6). Tasks like the PASAT, which tap a number of different cognitive processes including retrieval from short term memory, make it a sensitive discriminator of cognitive speed between brain damaged patients and controls, particularly when stimuli are presented more quickly (Litvan et al., 1988), a similar effect noted in the optic neuritis sample with brain lesions. Tests that were not time dependent, namely the Raven's matrices, failed to distinguish between the groups.

Studies of cognitive change

Studies investigating cognitive change over time in MS have adopted one of two strategies. The first has taken a cross-sectional approach with the patient sample stratified according to disease duration. The second method has been to follow patients longitudinally with serial measurements of various cognitive indices.

Cross-sectional studies

These have found little evidence to support a progression of deficits. Ivnik (1978a) studied 36 patients with MS divided into triads on the basis of the number of years they had MS symptoms (i.e. 1–5; 6–10; >10 years). The three groups were matched for sex, education, and age of onset of symptoms. No cognitive differences were found between the three groups and only in tests dependent on intact tactile perception did the group with the longer duration perform more poorly. Halligan et al. (1988) divided 60 MS patients into three equal groups with differing durations of illness (<5; 5–15; >15 years) and found that a mild decline in abstracting and memory functions were present in the group with the longest duration of illness. However, other cognitive functions were intact, and occupational and social functioning appeared unrelated to duration.

Although providing some pointers to a lack of correlation between cognitive decline and disease duration, the studies were unable to elucidate the nature of individual cognitive change. Although logistically easier to perform than longitudinal studies, they could, at best, supply indirect evidence of how cognition changes with time.

Longitudinal studies

Follow-up studies of patients with clinically isolated lesions
The study of patients with acute optic neuritis demonstrated that cognitive

abnormalities, not necessary clinically detectable, but rather demonstrable on detailed neuropsychological examination were present within weeks of the development of the earliest neurological symptoms. How these cognitive difficulties progressed as the disease evolved was the objective of Feinstein et al. (1992b), who undertook a follow-up cognitive, psychiatric and MRI study of Callanan's original cohort of CIL patients. Subjects were reassessed after a mean interval of $4\frac{1}{2}$ years (range 42 to 67 months), by which time the sample size had decreased to 44 because the passage of time and re-examination of medical records made it clear that four cases had been incorrectly diagnosed. Thus, one patient was rediagnosed as having motor neurone disease, another with a presenile dementia of the Alzheimer type and two patients were reassessed as having had MS at their index examination. Of the remaining 44 subjects, 35 (80%) were prepared to return to hospital and undergo a repeat battery of cognitive tests and a second brain MRI. Psychometric testing examined the following areas: IQ deficit, verbal and visual recognition memory, verbal recall memory, abstracting ability, visual and auditory attention and naming ability.

At follow-up, half the subjects had developed MS with two-thirds following a relapsing–remitting (RR) course and the remainder in a chronic–progressive (CP) phase. As a group, the MS patients' cognitive performance had deteriorated significantly only with respect to visual memory, but when a three-way comparison was undertaken, the patients with a chronic–progressive course were more impaired on tests of verbal recall memory and auditory attention. The CP patients were also significantly more depressed, although this could not account for their greater cognitive difficulties. However, the CP patients had a greater lesion load on MRI and this correlated significantly with the degree of cognitive impairment. A noticeable finding was the marked individual variability that characterized cognitive change. If the patient's disease status remained unchanged, i.e. CIL at follow-up, there had been no change in cognitive function or mood status. Similarly, even if the disease had progressed from CIL to relapsing–remitting MS, no significant cognitive decline was discernable. The critical variable that determined intellectual deterioration was the degree to which the brain total lesion load had increased (see Chapter 9).

Follow-up studies of patients with MS

Rapidly progressive dementia in which patients experience profound physical and mental deterioration over the course of a few months has been described. Bergin (1957) reported two such cases, both young women, in one of whom the diagnosis was made only at postmortem. Cognitive decline was inexorable and rapid, ending in death. Such reports are, however, rare.

An early study by Fink and Houser (1966) noted that MS patients often had great difficulty completing the performance subscale of the Wechsler Adult Intelligence Scale (WAIS). They therefore confined their 1-year longitudinal study to an analysis of verbal measures, and reported that poor performance on tests such as Digit Span and Similarities correlated inversely with physical disability, i.e. the greater the physical disability, the worse the verbal score. Notwithstanding this observation, an overall 4-point improvement in verbal IQ was found. A relative preservation of verbal skills at the expense of psychomotor performance was also noted by Ivnik (1978b) in a 3-year follow-up study of 14 patients with MS. Similarly, Canter (1951a, b), in a 6-month follow-up of 47 MS patients and 38 healthy controls noted that, while deterioration was present on all but two of the Wechsler–Bellevue Scales, it was again the performance IQ which was most affected.

In the first wide-ranging longitudinal study of cognitive change Filley et al. (1990) retested a group of 46 MS patients with the expanded Halsteid–Reitan Battery after an interval of 1 to 2 years. The study was significant because it took into account many factors omitted from earlier studies (i.e. disease course and exacerbations, physical disability ratings and disease duration). The sample was divided at the outset into three categories: stable relapsing–remitting, exacerbating relapsing–remitting and chronic–progressive. Although the latter group were initially more cognitively impaired, confirming Heaton et al.'s (1985) original observation on the same sample, disease course and disease exacerbation were not strongly predictive of cognitive change. Furthermore, group data did not reveal a significant cognitive decline, and a deterioration in performance was noted on only 6 of 36 test measures. In some cases, the scores on summary measures such as performance IQ improved, which was put down to the effects of practice. It was, however, difficult to judge these changes without recourse to comparisons with healthy control subjects, a major limitation of the study. Any conclusion that significant cognitive deterioration did not occur over a 1 to 2-year period would thus have been premature.

Subsequent longitudinal studies have incorporated control subjects and generally come up with confluent findings. Jennekens-Schinkel et al. (1990) found that, although MS patients as a group were initially more cognitively impaired than a healthy control group, three-quarters of their sample did not show further cognitive decline after a 4-year follow-up period. In some patients improvement occurred, but whether this was related to the effects of practice or to a direct improvement in brain function was less clear as neuroimaging had not been completed. The authors commented on some of the difficulties inherent in longitudinal studies of MS patients, and cautioned that psychomotor deterioration (such as a patient's ability to rapidly assess visual information and respond accordingly) was not commensurate with a deterioration in other cognitive areas. They concluded that cognitive change showed considerable individual variation. This was also characteristic of variables such as disease course and physical disability (see Chapter 1) confirming their unreliability as predictors of cognitive decline.

A similar conclusion was reached by Amato et al. (1995) in a 4-year follow-up study of 50 patients with recent onset MS and 70 healthy control subjects. Deficits in verbal memory and abstract reasoning in the MS group, present at the index assessment, had generally not progressed. However, some new deficits had become apparent, namely problems with word fluency and verbal comprehension. Once again, variables such as disease course, physical disability and duration of illness could not predict a patient's cognitive status, but the situation with respect to disease activity was more equivocal. Although no association was reported between the annual relapse rate and cognitive impairment, this variable measured the frequency, but not the severity of relapses and the result may thus have been misleading. Evidence that cognition can deteriorate as part of a clinical exacerbation, only to recover once neurological improvement occurs, has been reported in individual patients (Bieliauskas et al., 1980; Rozewicz et al., 1996).

The most compelling data demonstrating little cognitive change over the course of a year comes from Hohol et al. (1997) in a study of 44 patients that focused largely on serial MRI brain changes. Most patients underwent 20 brain MRIs in the course of a year and lesion volume and brain volumes were assessed using computer-automated, three-dimensional volumetric analysis. All subjects also completed a brief repeatable neuropsychological battery for MS at the beginning and the end of the study. No overall deterioration in cognition was observed. A decline in cognitive status occurred only in four patients (9%) and was associated with an increase in total lesion volume. In the remaining 40 patients, cognitive performance had either remained stable (48%) or improved (43%).

A final aspect to cognitive change needs to be considered, namely whether short-term fluctuations in cognitive ability occur in patients who experience a clinical relapse or who have MRI evidence of lesion activity. There is evidence from serial studies (Willoughby et al. 1989; Thompson et al., 1992) that new lesions detected by MRI are not always mirrored by new symptoms or changes in neurological examination. The poor correlation between physical disability and the extent of brain pathology may result from the presence of lesions in sites not capable of producing motor or sensory symptoms and conversely, physical disability may emanate from spinal cord pathology which would be missed by a scan confined to the brrain. In order to assess the possibility of short-term fluctuations in cognition, Feinstein et al. (1993) studied two patient groups, namely five patients with early relapsing–remitting disease and an equal number with benign MS. Each patient was individually matched with a healthy control in terms of age, sex, and premorbid IQ.

The testing protocol called for patients to undergo contrast-enhanced MRI, neurological examination (including EDSS ratings) and neuropsychological evaluation at 2-weekly (early RR MS) and monthly (benign MS) intervals. Apart from the Purdue Pegboard Test, all psychometric tests were computerized to remove or minimize a motor component to testing and confined primarily to tests of attention and information processing speed, as they were thought to be less affected by practice than are other aspects of cognition. In addition, to further minimize the effects of practice, parallel versions of tests were employed and all patients and controls were tested psychometrically on two separate occasions before their first MRI.

The results indicated that patients, as a group, performed more poorly than controls on all psychometric tests, although both groups tended to improve over the 6-month period at a comparable rate. In patients with a relatively stable lesion load throughout the 6 months of the study, no consistent changes in test performance were noted, other than those at-tributable to practice effects, i.e. performances improved. On the other hand, those patients in whom lesion load had significantly increased displayed less uniform results. Some exhibited decline in test performance while others did not. The individual matching of patient with healthy control highlighted the great individual variability in the performance of MS subjects, but by group-ing all scores together these individual differences were obscured.

The study contained a wealth of data and illustrated the complexity of documenting cognitive change over time in MS. Like other studies (Jen-nekens-Schinkel et al., 1990; Amato et al., 1996; Hohol et al., 1997), it supported the observation of considerable variation, not only between pa-tients, but also within the same patient over time. In this regard, the perform-ances of the healthy controls, although superior to the MS patients in terms of quicker speed of response and fewer errors made, also demonstrated considerable inter- and intra- subject variability. In the MS cohort, psychomotor tasks were the most sensitive in detecting cognitive change, in keeping with earlier observations (Ivnik, 1978b). However, the study also demonstrated the ability of MS patients to improve their performance over time at a rate that paralleled their healthy counterparts. This ability to benefit from practice was, in most paradigms, maintained for the duration of the study. Some patients managed to improve their cognitive performance, despite a deteriorating MRI picture, illustrating the strength of practice effects and suggesting that cognitive deficits in certain MS patients are, to some degree at least, open to remediation.

Summary

• Subtle evidence of cognitive change may occur in patients with clinically isolated lesions of the type seen in MS thereby predating the diagnosis of MS. Cognitive change is thus one of the earliest manifestations of demyelination.

- Medium-term follow-up studies have demonstrated that further cognitive deterioration occurs in an minority of patients and that considerable individual variation characterizes cognitive change over time.
- The critical variable that determines the rate and extent of cognitive change is the development of increased brain lesion load.
- Neurological deterioration, duration of symptoms and a chronic–progressive disease course are not reliable predictors of cognitive decline.
- The performance of MS patients on serial psychometric measures demonstrates their often considerable ability to improve performance with practice. This improvement may, as a group, parallel that of healthy subjects, although baseline group differences will be maintained.

References

Amato MP, Ponziani G, Pracucci G, Bracco L, Siracusa G, Amaducci L. (1995) Cognitive impairment in early-onset multiple sclerosis. *Archives of Neurology*, **52**, 168–72.

Bergin JD. (1957) Rapidly progressive dementia in disseminated sclerosis. *Journal of Neurology, Neurosurgery and Psychiatry*, **20**, 285–92.

Bieliauskas LA, Topel J, Huckman MS. (1980) Cognitive, neurologic and radiologic test data in a changing lesion pattern. *Journal of Clinical Neuropsychology*, **2**, 217–30.

Callanan MM, Logsdail SJ, Ron M, Warrington EK. (1989) Cognitive impairment in patients with clinically isolated lesions of the type seen in multiple sclerosis. *Brain*, **112**, 361–74.

Canter AH (1951a) Direct and indirect measures of psychological deficit in multiple sclerosis. Part I. *The Journal of General Psychology*, **44**, 3–25.

Canter AH. (1951b) Direct and indirect measures of psychological deficit in multiple sclerosis. Part II. *The Journal of General Psychology*, **44**, 27–50.

Feinstein A, Youl B, Ron M. (1992a) Acute optic neuritis. A cognitive and magnetic resonance imaging study. *Brain*, **115**, 1403–15.

Feinstein A, Kartsounis L. Miller D, Youl B, Ron M. (1992b) Clinically isolated lesions of the type seen in multiple sclerosis: a cognitive, psychiatric and MRI follow-up study. *Journal of Neurology, Neurosurgery and Psychiatry*, **55**, 869–76.

Feinstein A, Ron M, Thompson A.(1993) A serial study of psychometric and magnetic resonance imaging changes in multiple sclerosis. *Brain*, **116**, 569–602.

Filley CM, Heaton RK, Thompson LL, Nelson LM, Franklin GM. (1990) Effects of disease course on neuropsychological functioning. In *Neurobehavioural Aspects of Multiple Sclerosis*, ed. SM Rao. pp. 136–48. New York: Oxford University Press.

Fink SL, Houser HB. (1966) An investigation of physical and intellectual changes in multiple sclerosis. *Archives of Physical Medicine and Rehabilitation*, **2**, 56–61.

Francis DA, Compston DAS, Batchelor JR and McDonald WI. (1987) A reassessment of the risk of multiple sclerosis developing in patients with optic neuritis after extended follow-up. *Journal of Neurology, Neurosurgery and Psychiatry*, **50**, 758–65.

Halligan FR, Reznikoff M, Friedman HP, La Rocca NG. (1988) Cognitive dysfunction and change in multiple sclerosis. *Journal of Clinical Psychology*, **44**, 540–8.

Heaton RK, Nelson LM, Thompson DS, Burk JS, Franklin GM. (1985) Neuro-psychological findings in relapsing-remitting and chronic-progressive multiple sclerosis. *Journal of Consulting and Clinical Psychology*, **53**, 103–10.

Hohol MJ, Guttmann CRG, Orav J, Mackin GA, Kikinis R et al. (1997) Serial neuropsychological assessment and magnetic resonance imaging analysis in multiple sclerosis. *Archives of Neurology*, **54**, 1018–25.

Ivnik RJ. (1978a) Neuropsychological test performance as a duration of MS-related symptomatology. *The Journal of Clinical Psychiatry*, **46**, 304–12.

Ivnik RJ. (1978b) Neuropsychological stability in multiple sclerosis. *Journal of Consulting and Clinical Psychology*, **46**, 913–23.

Jennekens-Schinkel A, Laboyrie PM, Lanser JBK, van der Velde EA. (1990) Cognition in patients with multiple sclerosis after four years. *Journal of Neurological Sciences*, **99**, 229–47.

Litvan I, Grafman J, Vendrell P, Martinez JM. (1988) Slowed information processing in multiple sclerosis. *Archives of Neurology*, **45**, 281–5.

Lyon-Caen O, Jouvent R, Hauser S, Chaunu M-P, Benoit N, Widlöcher D, Lhermitte F. (1986) Cognitive function in recent onset demyelinating diseases. *Archives of Neurology*, **43**, 1138–41.

Rozewicz L, Langdon DW, Davie CA, Thompson A, Ron M. (1996) Resolution of left hemisphere cognitive dysfunction in multiple sclerosis with magnetic resonance correlates: a case report. *Cognitive Neuropsychiatry*, **1**, 17–25.

Thompson AJ, Miller D, Youl B et al. (1992) Serial gadolinium enhanced MRI in relapsing-remitting multiple sclerosis of varying disease duration. *Neurology (Cleveland)*, **42**, 60–3.

Willoughby EW, Grochowski E, Li DKB, Oger J, Kastrukoff LF, Paty DW. (1989) Serial magnetic resonance imaging scanning in multiple sclerosis: a second prospective study in relapsing–remitting patients. *Annals of Neurology*, **25**, 43–9.

8

Cognitive impairment in multiple sclerosis: detection, management and significance

With the recognition that cognitive impairment affects approximately 40% of patients with MS, new challenges have presented themselves. Among them is a need to accurately detect cognitive abnormalities in a time-efficient, cost-effective way. Almost three out of four patients with cognitive dysfunction will be missed during the routine neurological examination, indicating that neurological impairment is not a reliable predictor of deficits (Peyser et al., 1980). While there is no alternative to neuropsychological testing in this regard, the procedure is time-consuming, expensive and may not be readily available in many centres.

This has prompted a search for a brief, reliable and easy-to-score method for eliciting deficits that may also lend itself to repeat testing for documenting cognitive change over time. As a result, the efficacy of existing cognitive screening procedures, such as the Mini-Mental State Examination (Folstein et al., 1975) have been assessed in patients with MS, while efforts at developing new measures specifically targeting this population have gathered pace. This chapter will critically revue their effectiveness and comment on some of the difficulties in producing a cognitive scale directed primarily at the detection of subcortical pathology. One of the problems inherent in this search is that MS, unlike many other causes of dementia, is not invariably associated with progressive brain involvement and by extension, cognitive decline (Heaton et al., 1990). Thus, screening instruments must differentiate not only between dementia and health, but also between MS patients with, and without, cognitive difficulties. Adding to the challenge, cognitive dysfunction may be relatively mild and circumscribed and vary across individuals.

The chapter will conclude with a discussion of the clinical significance of cognitive impairment and a summary of the treatment options open to patients. One point should, however, be made early on. It is self-evident to state that, when discussing the possibility of cognitive decline with MS patients, considerable tact and sensitivity are called for. Many patients are young and may still be working. Many are in the process of coming to terms either with the diagnosis of MS or the loss of some neurological function. These factors alone demand psychological resilience. Adding the spectre of dementia may prove emotionally overwhelming. It may also prove unfounded. When confronting patients' fears on this score, the author's approach is to point out that the majority of MS patients ($\pm 60\%$) do *not* have cognitive decline and in those who do, deficits may be mild and non-progressive. At the same time, it is doing some patients a disservice to downplay deficits that are present. As this chapter will make clear, cognitive testing is not mandatory in every MS subject. It is up to the clinician to decide on the judicious use of this investigation according to the individual merits of each case. Guidelines in this regard are provided.

The mini-mental state examination

The Mini-Mental State Examination (MMSE) (Folstein et al., 1975) was developed to provide a quick, standardized method for assessing cognition. The test examines orientation to time and place, attention (serial subtractions or reverse spelling), short-term and secondary memory, constructional ability and language and the individual scores summed to give a total out of 30. Initially, a cut-off score of 20 was used to signify dementia (Folstein et al., 1975), but this has subsequently been raised to < 24 (De Paulo and Folstein, 1978). The MMSE takes approximately 5–10 minutes to complete, and is now widely used in a variety of clinical and research settings. Although not formulated for disorders predominantly involving subcortical white matter, the MMSE has been used to cognitively screen patients with MS, prompting queries about its validity.

Studies have found the MMSE helpful in a MS research setting, but a closer look at the raw data raises questions about the clinical usefulness of the results. In particular, the ability of cognitively impaired MS patients to frequently score well within the normal range suggests major deficiencies when the instrument is applied to this population. Huber et al. (1987) and Rao et al. (1991a) found statistically significant differences between patients with MS and healthy controls, but in both studies the mean MMSE scores for the MS samples were well above the cut-off point for dementia. Similarly, Rao et al. (1989) found that cognitively impaired MS patients had a significantly lower MMSE score than cognitively intact MS patients, but the means scores for both groups were again greater than 27. A similar situation pertains to another brief screening instrument, the Cognitive Capacity Screening Examination (CCSE) (Jacobs et al., 1977). This instrument assesses orientation, immediate and short-term memory (after a brief distraction), attention, calculation, delayed recall and verbal reasoning (similarities and opposites). Like the MMSE, a score out of 30 is obtained and anything less than 20 is considered impaired. Heaton et al. (1990) demonstrated that the CCSE was better able than the MMSE to differentiate MS patients from healthy controls, but scores on the CCSE were also within the upper normal range, thereby compromising clinical utility.

Despite these failings, the MMSE has remained a potentially attractive option to researchers and clinicians alike, due to its brevity and wide usage in a neurological setting. It has also stimulated a number of comparisons with other more comprehensive methods of cognitive assessment. Franklin et al. (1988) looked at the effectiveness of the MMSE versus a 45-minute, comprehensive neuropsychological battery in detecting cognitive impairment in a group of 60 patients with clinically definite, chronic–progressive MS. A cut-off point of 24 on the MMSE was used and no MS patient scored below this, although 83% of the same sample (60% when motor deficits were taken into account) were found to be impaired on the more detailed testing. Attempts to apply a different cut-off score to the MMSE based on results from the neuropsychological battery were equally problematic and managed to identify only 20% of the cognitively impaired sample.

Prompted by Franklin et al.'s (1988) demonstration of poor sensitivity, but cognizant of the need for brevity, Beatty and Goodkin (1990) investigated ways of improving the efficacy of the MMSE. A limited battery of cognitive tests were given to a sample of 85 MS patients evenly divided between a relapsing–remitting (RR) and chronic–progressive (CP) course. The tests included the Boston Naming Test (i.e. total number correct, uncued), The Wisconsin Card Sort Test (i.e. number of categories achieved out of 6), speed of information processing (measured either by a test of verbal fluency (FAS test) or the Symbol-Digit Modality Test(SDMT)) and various memory paradigms (i.e. recognition and recall for both short-term and remote memory). Dementia was defined as impairment (i.e. scores at or below the fifth percentile relative to healthy control subjects) on three of the four functions tested. In addition, a modified version of the MMSE, controlling for possible motor difficulties, was completed by all subjects.

The results confirmed the deficiencies of the MMSE when used in this population. Thus, of the 35 patients with a 100% MMSE score, 34% were impaired on the SDMT, 23.5% scored below the fifth percentile on the FAS test and a test of long-term recognition memory, while the percentage of patients demonstrating impaired performance on the remainder of the tests varied from 9.4% to 20%. With a MMSE score indicating dementia (i.e. < 24) all subjects were impaired on every cognitive test. Of the nine tests in the battery, the SDMT was found to be the most sensitive, followed by the WCST and a test of immediate recall. Most tellingly, a quarter of patients with a MMSE score in the normal range were impaired on all tests. Raising the cut-off score did not help either. A score of 27 still missed too many impaired individuals while a score of 28 produced an unacceptably high number of false positives.

Adding the Boston Naming Test or the SDMT to the MMSE, or increasing the number of recall items from 3 to 7, were suggested as ways to improve sensitivity. Of the three, the SDMT was the most sensitive and Beatty and

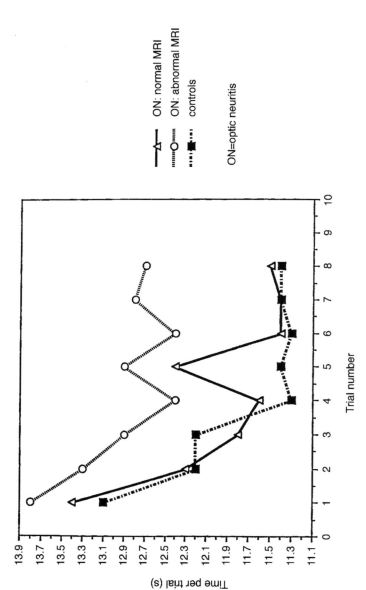

Fig. 8.1   Symbol–Digit Modality Test: optic neuritis and control group performances (Feinstein et al. 1992). By permission of Oxford University Press.

Goodkin (1990) advocate incorporating it in all screening procedures. The test, which takes only a few minutes to complete can be presented in a computerized form, thereby preventing difficulties with writing from obscuring true cognitive deficits. Feinstein et al. (1992) have demonstrated that the SDMT is a sensitive indicator of cognitive difficulties even in the prodromal phase of MS. Using a version of the paradigm that required subjects to match nine symbols with nine numbers over eight trials, the test was able to discriminate between healthy controls and optic neuritis patients with and without brain lesions (see Fig. 8.1).

Finally, the most comprehensive study of the MMSE in multiple sclerosis to date provides further compelling evidence that the instrument lacks sensitivity in detecting cognitive impairment (Swirsky-Sacchetti et al., 1992). The relationship of MMSE scores to a host of variables, such as brain lesion area on MRI, physical disability as measured by the EDSS (Kurtzke, 1983) and Scripps neurologic rating scale (Sipe et al., 1984) and cognition assessed by detailed neuropsychological testing, was investigated. The neuropsychological tests were chosen to minimize a sensorimotor component and included indices of abstract/conceptual reasoning, language, memory, visuoperceptual skills and processing speed. A subject was considered demented if the performance was impaired relative to normative data on 50% or more of the 11 neuropsychological tests.

The mean MMSE score for the 56 MS patients was 26.51(sd=3.51) and 16% of patients performed below the cut-off point of 24. The 72% false negative rate fell to 9% if the cut-off was raised to 27/30, but false positives then rose to an unacceptable high 30%. The MMSE was the only cognitive index that did not correlate significantly with total lesion area in the brain. Significant correlations, however, were present between scores on the MMSE and the EDSS and Scripps scales, suggesting the MMSE may be more reflective of overall disease severity, including physical disability, than a measure of subtle cognitive impairment. The study underscored the point made by earlier reports that the MMSE was not a suitable cognitive screening measure in MS because it contained too few items able to quantify cognitive aspects of a subcortical, white matter disease.

Other brief screening procedures

In a frequently cited study Rao et al. (1991a) reported that 43% of a community-based sample of MS patients had cognitive impairment. They arrived at this conclusion using a battery of 22 neuropsychological tests and then went on to determine which of the tests were the most sensitive detectors of impairment. The result was the development of a cognitive screening measure that takes 15–20 minutes to complete and comprises four tests; the Consistent Long-Term Retrieval from Selective Reminding Test (CLTR), the Total Recall from 7/24 Spatial Recall Test (7/24), the Controlled Oral Word Association Test (COWAT) and the Paced Auditory Serial Addition Test (PASAT), the latter using stimuli presented at 3 seconds and 2 seconds. Taking impairment on any two tests as a sign of cognitive dysfunction, the brief battery had a 71% sensitivity and a 94% specificity, a considerable improvement compared to the MMSE. Furthermore, 15 alternative, equivalent versions of the tests were developed for longitudinal research purposes, such as studying the natural history of cognitive change and possible cognitive responses in treatment trials.

To investigate the effectiveness of a cognitive screening procedure in a serial setting, Bever et al. (1995) used the Brief Repeatable Neuropsychological Battery (the original four tests in Rao et al.'s battery plus the Symbol-Digit Modality Test) and tested a group of 19 MS patients at 60 day intervals for 3 months. In keeping with longitudinal studies using more comprehensive cognitive batteries (see Chapter 7), they noted individual variability over time and the ability of patients to benefit from practice. This finding was replicated by Hohol et al. (1997) in a serial MRI study that used the four-item Rao et al. battery to assess cognition at entry to the study and after completion, 1 year later. Not only did the brief battery detect cognitive change, but results correlated significantly with changes in brain lesion load, thereby supplying a further marker of validity.

Although an improvement on the MMSE, Rao et al.'s procedure has been criticized for the high false negative rate and the narrow range of cognitive abilities assessed. Attempting to overcome these limitations, Basso et al. (1996) developed a 35–50 minute cognitive screen that retained some of the cognitive indices recommended by Rao and colleagues, but added others. Thus, both batteries contain measures of auditory attention (Seashore Rhythm Test (Basso et al.) versus PASAT (Rao et al.)), verbal fluency (COWAT in both) and verbal learning (Logical Memory Saving Score (Basso et al.) versus Consistent Long-Term Retrieval from the Selective Reminding Test (Rao et al.)). However, the Rao battery included another measure of memory, namely a non-verbal short-term recall test while Basso et al. included tests of graphesthesia and astereognosis. The latter are surprising inclusions given the infrequency with which similar abnormalities have been reported in MS patients. Nevertheless their addition contributed to a screening procedure with a 100% sensitivity and a 80% specificity. Thus, in relation to the Rao battery, more cognitively impaired patients are detected at the expense of over-diagnosis. Whether this is a meaningful improvement depends on your perspective. The advantages of improved detection are self-evident, but false positives bring their own potential problems, such as engendering anxiety and depression in a group that is known to be prone to mood disorders. Furthermore, the Basso battery takes longer to administer which may offset any advantage. Indeed, the 35–50 minute duration places it alongside other intermediate length instruments.

Intermediate length cognitive screening procedures

What is meant by 'intermediate' is arbitrary, but one safe definition is to include all those batteries whose length of administration falls between the day long duration as typified by the Expanded Halstead–Reitan Battery on the one hand and brief measures such as the MMSE (5–10 minutes) and the Rao et al. battery (±20 minutes) on the other. A number of such intermediate length procedures have been developed ranging from an 18–item battery (Heaton et al., 1990) that takes approximately 45 minutes, to a core battery of neuropsychological tests recommended by the National Multiple Sclerosis Society that may take up to 2 hours (Peyser et al., 1990). The advantage to this approach, compared to the brief screening measures, is that it supplies a more comprehensive analysis of a patient's cognitive deficiencies and strengths, both of which are important when it comes to planning remediation. This point deserves emphasizing. While researchers may disagree on the exact composition of what constitutes the most effective screening instrument, they all concur that within a clinical setting, an important function of screening patients is to identify those who may require a more comprehensive assessment, without which it is impossible to gain a complete understanding of the scope and degree of the intellectual difficulties.

Indications for comprehensive testing

Under what circumstances should cognitive testing be completed and how should this be done? Does the patient require a brief or a comprehensive assessment? How should the patient be approached with a view to suggesting an assessment, and when completed, how should the results be presented back to the patient? Answers to some of these will be dictated by circumstances. For example, not every neurologist will have access to a neuropsychologist who can undertake the testing and for many patients, such a service may not be affordable. However, most larger centres are able to provide psychometric testing and the advantages and drawbacks to recommending an assessment have to be carefully weighted.

Before deciding to proceed with neuropsychological testing, the physician has to weight the options carefully. Some patients who are newly diagnosed with MS may find the thought of possible (or confirmed) cognitive dysfunction overwhelming, whereas to the patient with longstanding disease, confirmation of deficits may come as a relief and explain years of self-perceived, but poorly understood intellectual difficulties.

A decade of research has provided certain pointers to whether cognitive function should be investigated or not. Most MS patients will have had a brain MRI as part of their initial work-up. Given that cognitive dysfunction is significantly associated with cerebral involvement, a brain MRI with a large lesion load and/or significant atrophy of the corpus callosum or generalized cortical atrophy should alert the neurologist to, at the very least, inquire about cognitive difficulties. The importance of listening to what family members have to say is emphasized, because MS patients, with possible impairment in metamemory (see Chapter 6) may not be the best judge of their own difficulties. The presence of frontal release signs, in particular those affecting the lower limbs, are also a predictor of associated cognitive dysfunction (Franklin et al., 1990). Under these circumstances, screening patients as a preliminary procedure would be indicated.

Some further guidelines about when to test and whether to use a modest screening test or proceed to more detailed testing have been provided by Franklin et al. (1990). Indications for neuropsychological assessment include the patient who complains that cognitive difficulties affect functioning at home or at work, the patient whose employer reports a fall-off in work performance, the patient seeking vocational counselling to obtain employment matched to his or her disability, the rehabilitation patient in whom suspected cognitive dysfunction may be impeding the progress of treatment, the patient entering a treatment trial and a pretreatment cognitive baseline is required and the patient with a treatment resistant depression who may initially have been diagnosed with pseudodementia (see Chapter 6). Furthermore should any of these situations arise in the context of an MRI displaying a heavy lesion load or significant atrophy, either generalized or confined to the corpus callosum, the argument for neuropsychological testing becomes even more compelling.

Conversely, some clear contraindications to testing include the patient who denies cognitive difficulties (without objective evidence to dispute his or her claim) and the patient who is significantly physically disabled, in a low demand environment and in whom cognitive assessment is unlikely to furnish fresh insights or lead to a change in patient care.

Counselling the patient pre- and post-testing is important in dealing with the attendant anxieties and with the implications pertaining to the findings.

Management strategies

Little has been written about therapy for cognitive difficulties in MS. Approaches may be divided into two broad categories, namely restorative or compensatory (Sohlberg and Mateer, 1989). Restorative refers to a process whereby cognitive deficits are identified and specific, remedial therapies introduced with the aim of increasing performance in that area. In contrast to this, compensatory strategies do not try to bring about a recovery of function. Rather, attempts are made at maximizing those abilities an individual retains. It is the latter approach that has received the most attention in MS.

Compensatory strategies

Before describing this particular form of therapy, it is of note that, in those MS patients who perceive themselves as cognitively impaired, the strategies that are spontaneously adopted are compensatory in nature. Thus, Sullivan et al. (1990) reported that the use of an external memory aid such as a notepad was frequently employed by patients.

Compensatory strategies are based on three tenets: structuring, scheduling and recording. The underlying principle is to bring as much structure and stability to the patients environment. This, in turn, ensures a measure of predictability, thereby reducing demands on planning, organization and memory (Sullivan et al., 1989). A first step in the process is to assess the individuals current cognitive strengths and weakness through neuro-psychological testing. An estimate of premorbid IQ via the vocabulary subtest on the WAIS is useful as an approximate marker of what the patient was capable of intellectually prior to the onset of MS. An assessment of the patient's environment is also mandatory, since this provides information on the daily demands confronting the MS patient. With this information, the therapist can identify those areas of daily functioning that are most affected by cognitive difficulties, and these are discussed with the patient before a specific plan is implemented. Consultations with family at this point are helpful because any changes that need to be implemented may require their cooperation.

Once this stage is complete, implementation can begin. Thus, the use of a day calendar as an aide mémoire for patients with memory difficulties could be tried. It is not enough just to suggest patients go out and buy the day calendar as they will also require help in deciding when, and what kinds of, information need to be recorded (Sullivan et al., 1989). When it comes to difficulties with planning and organization, be they at home or at work, attempts at manipulating the environment to provide greater structure could be tried. Thus, using a day planner, patients are reminded that a specified task should be carried out at a set time each day, using items that should always kept in the same place. Depending on a patient's cognitive ability, this structure may be applied to factors ranging from work-related tasks to the more mundane activities of daily living such as meal preparation, grocery shopping, cleaning, transportation and personal safety issues (Bennett et al., 1991).

Remedial strategies

Unlike another neurological disorder such as head injury (Grafman, 1984), little attention has focused on remedial strategies in MS patients. The reasons probably relate to the nature of cognitive dysfunction in MS. Unlike stroke and head injury, where the insult is sudden and is followed by a period of expected, albeit variable recovery, MS-related cognitive change follows an altogether different course. The onset may be insidious, and deterioration, if it is to occur over time, is unlikely to be interrupted by periods of cognitive improvement. For this reason, compensation strategies in MS are considered more useful (Minden and Moes, 1990).

Despite a preference for compensatory approaches, remediation has been tried in MS patients. A process of graded practice for improving memory, using computer-run programmes has been implemented in at least one MS rehabilitation setting, but results have yet to be reported (LaRocca, 1990). In a study that randomly assigned 40 MS patients to one of two groups, i.e. remediation plus compensation versus non-specific, diffuse mental stimulation, the former was found to be more effective, with improvements reported in some memory functions after a 6-month follow-up (Jonsson et al., 1993). Such results, while encouraging, need replication.

Irrespective of the approach used, attempts at cognitive rehabilitation should not take place in isolation. It should be but one part of a comprehensive treatment strategy that begins the moment MS is diagnosed. Such an approach which focuses primarily on the patient, but includes family members when relevant, embraces not only cognitive strategies, but also includes treatment for neurological symptoms (e.g. the interferon compounds), psychopathology (antidepressant and anxiolytic medication, psychotherapy) and help for psychosocial difficulties.

Medication to help cognition

The importance of not missing the diagnosis of pseudodementia has been dealt with earlier in this chapter, and treatment requires the use of antidepressant medication. In addition, there is also the possibility of drug therapy directed at physical disability having beneficial effects on cognitive functioning as well. One such drug is 4-aminopyridene, a potassium channel blocker which may reduce physical disability in some MS patients (van Diemen et al., 1992). To assess the effects on cognition, Smits et al. (1994) undertook a randomized, double blind, placebo-controlled, crossover study in 20 MS patients using serial neuropsychological testing. Although there was a trend for patients to show cognitive improvement on some tests, the results were not promising.

Nevertheless, a number of potentially effective drugs for the treatment of MS (interferon beta-1b, beta-1a) have subsequently come on the market. Their effects on cognition have yet to be determined. If these drugs can reduce brain lesion load or the extent of brain lesion enhancement (a marker of disease activity), they offer the possibility of not only arresting cognitive decline, but also reversing some of the impairment. Brief, repeatable neuropsychological batteries are now included in MS drug trials and the results awaited.

Cognitive therapy to help cognition

Although cognitive therapy has been used to treat patients with depression in a psychiatric setting and has been applied only in a limited fashion to depressed MS subjects (see Chapter 2), Rodgers et al. (1996) have shown that the treatment modality may have some beneficial effects on certain aspects of cognition too. Thus, after 24 weeks of therapy, improvement in verbal learning and memory, but not vocabulary, information processing speed and visual acuity were noted in a small number of patients. However, depression scores also lessened with therapy and it is unclear to what extent the cognitive improvement was independent of the change in mood. Nevertheless, the significance of the findings coupled with the knowledge that treatment, unlike medication, is devoid of troubling side effects, emphasizes the need for replication in a larger sample.

The clinical significance of cognitive impairment

The best evidence that cognitive dysfunction exerts an adverse effect on MS patients' social functioning comes from Rao et al.'s (1991b) community study of 100 patients, who were almost evenly divided on the basis of detailed neuropsychological testing into cognitively intact and impaired groups. The two groups, who were closely matched on demographic characteristics and factors such as duration of illness, disease course, physical disability and the percentage taking medication, were then compared across a number of different parameters that included measures of physical disability, an occupational therapy assessment, self-report measures of depression, anxiety and sickness related disability and an informant's (relative or friend) rating of the subject's emotional adjustment. The cognitively impaired patients were found to be at a considerable social disadvantage with difficulties spanning work, relationships, vocational activities, sexual function and activities of daily living. The study was, however, cross-sectional, and the authors therefore cautioned against drawing direct etiological inferences. Follow-up data supporting these conclusions comes from Amato et al. (1995) who also noted that cognitive difficulties impinge adversly on patients' everyday func-tion-ing, even early on in the disease process.

Summary

- The routine neurological examination and mental state assessment will miss detecting cognitive dysfunction in the majority of MS patients, hence the need for sensitive, brief screening procedures.
- The Mini-Mental State Examination is not useful in screening patients with multiple sclerosis for cognitive impairment.
- A screening procedure encompassing four cognitive tests has been developed by Rao et al. (1991a), that has good sensitivity and specificity, takes 15–20 minutes to complete and may be used in serial studies, given that parallel versions of the tests are available.
- Cognitive batteries of intermediate length (45–60 minutes) have also been developed to provide more detailed information on a patient's deficits and residual strengths.
- There are situations in which a comprehensive neuropsychological assessment, such as the Halsteid–Reitan Battery, may be required. Indications for this are provided in the text. The clinician is therefore, faced with a choice of options when it comes to exploring suspected cognitive dysfunction, and the individual circumstances of the patient will determine which route to go.
- Rehabilitation generally follows a compensatory, as opposed to a remedial, approach. The aim is to enhance a patient's occupational or psychosocial functioning (both, if relevant) by utilizing residual cognitive strengths and planning around them.
- There are empirical data demonstrating that cognitive dysfunction exerts an adverse effect on a patient's quality of life in many different spheres, ranging from the workplace to relationships to such basic aspects as the activities of daily living.

References

Amato MP, Gluseppina P, Bracco L, Siracusa G, Amaducci L. (1995) Cognitive impairment in early-onset multiple sclerosis: patterns, predictors, and impact on everyday life in a 4 year follow-up. *Archives of Neurology*, **52**, 168–72.

Basso MR, Beason-Hazen S, Lynn J, Rammohan K, Bornstein RA. (1996) Screening for cognitive dysfunction in multiple sclerosis. *Archives of Neurology*, **53**, 980–4.

Beatty WW, Goodkin DE. (1990) Screening for cognitive impairment in multiple sclerosis. An evaluation of the Mini-Mental State Examination. *Archives of Neurology*, **47**, 297–301.

Bennett T, Dittmar C, Raubach S. (1991) Multiple Sclerosis: cognitive deficits and rehabilitation strategies. *Cognitive Rehabilitation*, **September/October**, 18–23.

Bever CT, Grattan L, Panitch HS, Johnson KP. (1995) A brief repeatable battery of neuropsychological tests for multiple sclerosis: a preliminary serial study. *Multiple Sclerosis*, **1**, 165–9.

DePaulo JR, Folstein MF. (1978) Psychiatric disturbance in neurological patients: detection, recognition, and hospital course. *Annals of Neurology*, **4**, 225–8.

Feinstein A, Youl B, Ron M. (1992) Acute optic neuritis. A cognitive and magnetic resonance imaging study. *Brain*, **115**, 1403–15.

Folstein MF, Folstein SE, McHugh PR. (1975) Mini-Mental State: a practical method for grading the cognitive state of patients for the clinician. *Journal of Psychiatric Research*, **12**, 189–98.

Franklin GM, Heaton RK, Nelson LM, Filley CM, Seibert C. (1988) Correlation of neuropsychological and MRI findings in chronic–progressive multiple sclerosis. *Neurology*, **38**, 1826–9.

Franklin GM, Nelson LM, Heaton RK, Filley CM. (1990) Clinical perspectives in the identification of cognitive impairment. In *Neurobehavioural Aspects of Multiple Sclerosis*, ed. SM Rao, pp. 161–74. New York: Oxford University Press.

Grafman J. (1984) Memory assessment and remediation. In *Behavioural Assessment and Rehabilitation of the Traumatically Brain Damaged*, ed. BA Edelstein, ET Couture pp. 151–89. New York: Plenum Press.

Heaton RK, Thompson LL, Nelson LM, Filley CM, Franklin GM. (1990) Brief and intermediate length screening of neuropsychological impairment in multiple sclerosis. in *Neurobehavioural Aspects of Multiple Sclerosis*, ed. SM Rao. pp 149–60. New York: Oxford University Press.

Hohol MJ, Guttmann CRG, Orav J et al. (1997) Serial neuropsychological assessment and magnetic resonance imaging analysis in multiple sclerosis. *Archives of Neurology*, **54**, 1018–25.

Huber SJ, Paulson GW, Shuttleworth EC et al. (1987) Magnetic resonance imaging correlates of dementia in multiple sclerosis. *Archives of Neurology*, **44**, 732–6.

Jacobs JW, Bernhard MR, Delgado A, Strain JJ. (1977) Screening for organic mental symptoms in the medically ill. *Annals of Internal Medicine*, **86**, 40–6.

Jonsson A, Korfitzen EM, Heltberg A, Ravnborg MH, Byskoz-Ottosen E. (1993) Effects of neuropsychological treatment in patients with multiple sclerosis. *Acta Neurologica Scandinavica*, **88**, 394–400.

Kurtzke JF. (1983) Rating neurologic impairment in multiple sclerosis: an expanded disability rating scale. *Neurology*, **33**, 1444–52.

LaRocca N. (1990) Management of neurobehavioural dysfunction. A rehabilitation perspective. In *Neurobehavioural Aspects of Multiple Sclerosis*, ed. SM Rao. pp 215–29. New York: Oxford University Press.

Minden S, Moes E. (1990) Management of neurobehavioural dysfunction. A psychiatric perspective. In *Neurobehavioural Aspects of Multiple Sclerosis*, ed. SM Rao pp. 230–50. New York: Oxford University Press.

Peyser JM, Edwards KR, Poser CM, Filskov SB. (1980) Cognitive function in patients with multiple sclerosis. *Archives of Neurology*, **37**, 577–9.

Peyser JM Rao SM, LaRocca NG, Kaplan E. (1990) Guidelines for neuropsychological research in multiple sclerosis. *Archives of Neurology*, **47**, 94–7.

Rao SM, Leo GJ, Bernardin L, Unverzagt F. (1991a) Cognitive dysfunction in multiple sclerosis. 1. Frequency, patterns, and prediction. *Neurology*, **41**, 685–91.

Rao SM, Leo GJ, Ellington L, Nauertz T, Bernardin L, Unverzagt F. (1991b) Cognitive dysfunction in multiple sclerosis. 11. Impact on employment and social functioning. *Neurology*, **41**, 692–6.

Rao SM, Leo GJ, Haughton VM, St. Aubin-Faubert P, Bernardin L. (1989) Correlation of magnetic resonance imaging and neuropsychological testing in multiple sclerosis. *Neurology*, **39**, 161–6.

Rodgers D, Khoo K, MacEachen M, Oven M, Beatty WW. (1996) Cognitive therapy for multiple sclerosis: A preliminary study. *Alternative Therapies in Health and Medicine*, **2**, 70–4.

Sipe JC, Knobler RL, Braheny SL, Rice GP, Panitch HS, Oldstone MB. (1984) A neurologic rating scale (NRS) for use in multiple sclerosis. *Neurology*, **34**, 1368–72.

Smits RCF, Emmen HH, Bertelsmann FW, Kulig BM, van Loenen AC, Polman CH. (1994) The effects of 4-aminopyridine on cognitive function in patients with multiple sclerosis: a pilot study. *Neurology*, **44**, 1701–5.

Sohlberg M, Mateer C. (1989) *Introduction to Cognitive Rehabilitation. Theory and Practice.* New York: Guildford.

Sullivan MJL, Dehoux E, Buchanan DC. (1989) An approach to cognitive rehabilitation in multiple sclerosis. *Canadian Journal of Rehabilitation*, **3**, 77–85.

Sullivan MJL, Edgley K, Dehoux E. (1990) A survey of multiple sclerosis. Part 1: Perceived cognitive problems and compensatory strategy use. *Canadian Journal of Rehabilitation*, **4**, 99–105.

Swirsky-Sacchetti T, Field HL, Mitchell DR et al. (1992) The sensitivity of the Mini-Mental State Examination in the white matter dementia of multiple sclerosis. *Journal of Clinical Psychology*, **48**, 779–86.

van Diemen, HAM, Polman CH, van Dongen TMMM et al. (1992) The effect of 4-aminopyridine on clinical signs in multiple sclerosis: a randomised, placebo-controlled, double-blind, cross-over study. *Annals of Neurology*, **32**, 123–30.

9

Neuroimaging correlates of cognitive dysfunction

This chapter will review evidence from structural and functional imaging studies and their attempts at correlating observed abnormalities with evidence of cognitive dysfunction. The emphasis is on Nuclear Magnetic Resonance imaging, in particular Magnetic Resonance Imaging (MRI), as this technique has the greatest sensitivity in visualizing MS plaques in the brain. It is no coincidence that the renewed interest shown by researchers in the neurobehavioural sequelae of MS dates from the advent of MRI as a research and clinical tool in the early 1980s. MRI provided a window into the brain of MS patients and offered an unprecedented opportunity to delineate the cerebral correlates of cognitive dysfunction. With the new-found, improved ability to visualize cerebral white matter in vivo, MRI has also provided fresh insights into the understanding of the concept of subcortical dementia. Another aspect to NMR technology, namely spectroscopy has more recently been applied to the study of MS, and the results of a preliminary study relating to cognition will be discussed. The chapter concludes with a review of the role of functional neuroimaging pertaining to MS and cognition.

Computerized axial tomography

Abnormalities on Computerized Axial Tomography (CT) in the brains of patients with MS were first reported in the mid-1970s (Warren et al., 1976; Glydensted, 1976). Although high resolution scanners, contrast enhancement and delayed scanning have all led to greater sensitivity in detecting MS lesions (Spiegel et al., 1985), the yield is still low compared to that of MRI (Young et al., 1981). It is nevertheless of value in demonstrating sulcal widening and ventricular dilatation, usually present in well-established, severe disease. Depending on the sample under study, these abnormalities have been found in 20–60% of MS subjects (Rao, 1990).

Given the lack of sensitivity of CT in detecting specific MS pathology, it is not surprising that correlations between imaging and cognitive measurements have been weak. No study has attempted to correlate the extent of lesion involvement in the brain with cognitive abnormalities, preferring to concentrate on parameters of cerebral atrophy instead. Brooks et al. (1984) estimated intellectual decline as the discrepancy between full-scale IQ

(WAIS) and a premorbid estimate based on reading test scores. They found, in their 13 patients, a strong association between IQ deficits and generalized cerebral atrophy. Rabins et al. (1986) similarly noted an inverse relationship between ventricular–brain ratio (VBR) and scores on the Mini-Mental State Examination, a course estimate of cognitive impairment.

In a more comprehensive study of CT and cognition, Rao et al. (1985) investigated 47 patients with chronic–progressive MS on tests of verbal and visuospatial learning and memory. Sulcal measurements were discarded as unreliable, and attention focused on the ventricular system. Variable degrees of ventriculomegaly were found in 60% of subjects and correlated with indices of cognitive decline. In particular, third ventricle width was the most sensitive CT indicator of intellectual and memory deficits. However, subsequent reanalysis of their data using improved measurement techniques failed to replicate this finding and led Rao (1990) to conclude that generalized and not just third ventricular enlargement was associated with cognitive decline.

The use of CT in MS has largely been superseded by MRI, and it is generally only in centres without ready access to MRI that CT scanning still takes place. The reasons are that comparisons between MRI and CT in MS have shown that the former detects many more lesions (Young et al., 1981) and, in cases where the diagnosis cannot be made with clinical criteria alone, MRI significantly increases the diagnostic yield over CT (Paty et al., 1988a). A comparison of the sensitivity of CT and MRI, the latter with and without contrast enhancement, in detecting MS brain lesions is shown in Figs. 9.1 (*a*), (*b*) and (*c*).

Magnetic resonance imaging

Monographs on magnetic resonance imaging (MRI) are available (Young, 1984; Andrew et al., 1990) and the reader looking for a detailed description of the principles and techniques is directed to them. However, a brief explanation is included to set in place the clinical–MRI correlations that follow.

Technique

MRI is a technique whereby images of objects, such as the brain, are created using nuclear magnetic resonance. In body tissues, before the application of a magnetic field, the magnetic moments of the protons (^1H) are randomly aligned and have zero net magnetization (M_0). When an external field is applied (e.g. produced by the magnet of the MRI imaging system), the individual magnetic moments align parallel or antiparallel with the applied

(a)

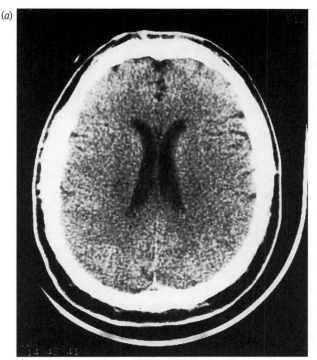

Fig 9.1.   A comparison of CT, MRI and contrast-enhanced (gadolinium-DTPA) MRI in one patient with MS. The CT and two MRI scans were performed within a day of each other and the sequences shown here are at the same anatomical level.
(a) Axial CT scan without evidence of MS plaques.

magnetic field. There are slightly more parallel than antiparallel protons, resulting in a slight net magnetization.

In a static magnetic field, the energy required to stimulate or excite the low energy parallel protons to higher energy antiparallel protons is supplied by electromagnetic radiofrequency (RF) waves. When radio waves of the right frequency are passed through the sample, some parallel protons will absorb energy and be excited to a higher energy state in the antiparallel direction. The amount of energy required to flip a proton from a parallel to an antiparallel orientation (and thus a higher energy state) is dependent on the strength of the magnetic field. The high energy protons are then observed as they return (relax) to their low energy state. In doing so, they emit electromagnetic energy of the same frequency as the RF source, and which is detected using a sensitive radio receiver. This is the signal that eventually generates the image to be viewed. The size or magnitude of the signal is

(b)

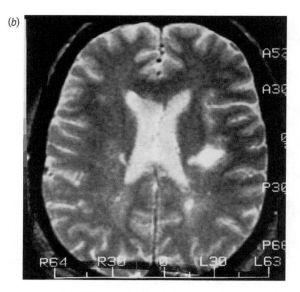

Fig 9.1(b).   Axial MRI scan (spin echo) in the same patient, showing lesions of varying sizes in both hemispheres.

(c)

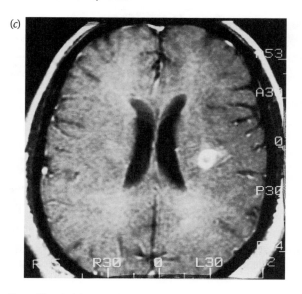

Fig 9.1(c).   Axial T_1-weighted gadolinium-DTPA-enhanced MRI scan, demonstrating the presence of a single, discrete contrast enhanced lesion corresponding with one of the plaques shown on the previous T_2-weighted (spin echo) image. Note that the other lesions shown in Fig. 9.1(b) are no longer visible.

Table 9.1 T_1 and T_2 MRI, CT and X-ray characteristics of normal tissue

	MR T_1	MR T_2	CT (X-ray)
Cortical bone	Very hypointense	Very hypointense	Very high density
Air	Very hypointense	Very hypointense	Very low density
Fat	Very hyperintense	Hypointense	Very low density
Water	Hypointense	Hyperintense	Low density
Brain	Grey matter=grey White matter=white	Intermediate (isointense)	Intermediate

proportional to the number of protons (proton density) in the tissue under study.

In principle, the procedure is confined to those nuclei that possess an odd number of either protons, neutrons or both, e.g. ^{1}H, ^{13}C, ^{19}F, ^{23}Na and ^{31}P, although, in practice, imaging is carried out on ^{1}H nuclei (protons) because of their high concentration (principally in water) and high nuclear magnetic resonance sensitivity.

T_1 and T_2-weighted images

Three principal properties of a substance can be measured, namely density of nuclear species (e.g. protons) and two relaxation times (T_1 and T_2). 'Relaxation time' refers to the time required for the net tissue magnetization vectors to come to equilibrium in a static external magnetic field. In the absence of an applied radiofrequency, transverse magnetization decays exponentially towards zero with a time constant T_2 and the longitudinal magnetization returns exponentially towards the equilibrium value M_0 with a characteristic time constant T_1. Relaxation times supply valuable information concerning the physical state of a sample and can detect pathological changes in tissues that appear macroscopically normal. Their values increase as the amount of free water in the sample increases, as in edema.

By varying the scanning parameters, i.e. using combinations of radio frequency pulses, a predominantly T_1 or proton density or T_2 -weighted image can be obtained. The different physical properties of normal (e.g. air, fat, etc) and abnormal (infarct, blood, tumour, MS plaque) tissue ensures that their appearance may be differentiated (Tables 9.1 and 9.2). In general, a T_1 -weighted image displays cerebral anatomy well, whereas a T_2 -weighted image is superior for detecting pathology, such as MS plaques. An useful intermediate scan, with characteristics between a T_1- and T_2 -weighted scan, is a proton density weighted sequence in which the CSF (water) shows up

Table 9.2 T_1 and T_2 CT and X-ray characteristics of abnormal tissue

	MR T_1	MR T_2	CT (X-ray)	Contrast enhancement[a]
Infarct	Hypointense	Hyperintense	Low density	Subacute
Blood	Very hyperintense[b]	Very hyperintense[b]	High density	No
Tumour	Hypointense	Hyperintense	Low density[c]	Yes
MS plaque	Hypointense	Hyperintense	Low density[d]	Acute

[a] enhancement signifies breakdown of the blood–brain barrier. Contrast used for MR is gadolinium-DTPA and for CT is iodinated material.
[b] blood appears bright unless very fresh or very old.
[c] tumour may appear hyperintense if calcified or hemorrhagic.
[d] MS plaque may appear isodense on CT, hence making detection difficult.

(a)

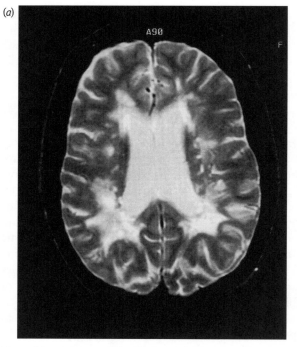

Fig. 9.2(a).   Axial T_2-weighted (spin echo) MRI scan, demonstrating extensive periventricular lesions typical of MS.

dark (hypointense), thereby offsetting the hyperintense MS plaque and allowing for better periventricular lesion–CSF discrimination (Figs. 9.2 (a), (b) and (c)).

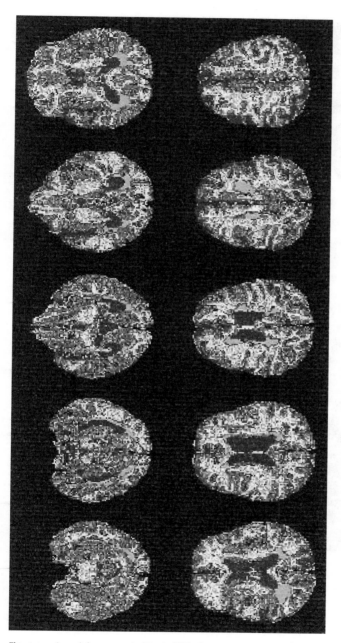

Fig. 9.4. An axial, segmented brain MRI of a 45-year-old woman with secondary progressive MS of 10 years' duration. The computerized brain segmentation (generated from T$_2$-weighted and proton density images) delineates four discrete areas: grey matter (dark grey), white matter (white), MS plaque (yellow) and CSF (dark blue).

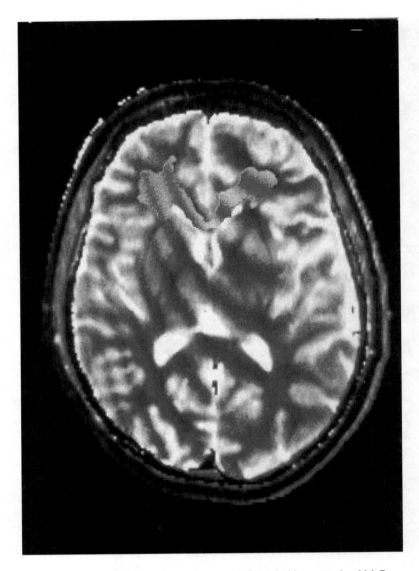

Fig. 9.8.   A demarcated area of normal appearing frontal white matter in which T_1 relaxation times were found to be abnormal, correlating with indices of cognitive impairment.

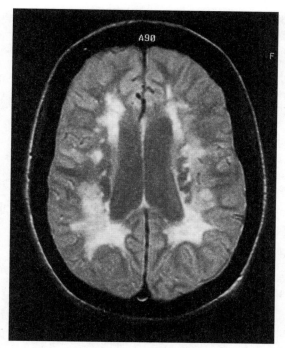

Fig. 9.2(*b*).   Axial proton density (spin echo) MRI scan in the same patient, at the same anatomical plane. Note how the CSF now appears hypointense (dark).

Magnetic resonance imaging in MS

Magnetic resonance imaging (MRI) is a highly sensitive technique for demonstrating brain lesions in patients with MS. Abnormalities are present in virtually all patients with clinically definite MS (Miller et al., 1988), the position of MRI lesions correlating with plaques seen at postmortem (Ormerod et al., 1987). The characteristic pattern is one of multifocal white matter lesions, the majority situated adjacent to the lateral ventricles.

Prolonged T_1 and T_2 relaxation times in MS patients compared to healthy controls (Ormerod et al., 1986) or those with systemic lupus erythematosus (Miller et al., 1989) have been noted, while patients with clinically isolated lesions (e.g. optic neuritis) tend to occupy an intermediate position between MS patients and healthy controls (Ormerod et al., 1986). The reasons for these changes are not entirely clear, but probably reflect the presence of microscopic abnormalities. such as perivascular inflammation, in the normal appearing white matter (Allen et al., 1981).

Although MRI has proved invaluable in providing a window to the brain in MS, it is not without limitations. Small, demyelinating lesions may escape detection because of restrictions on spatial resolution, although this problem

(c)

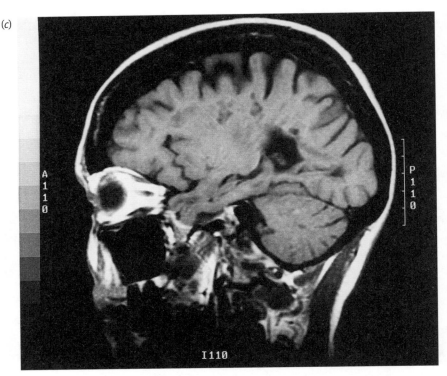

Fig. 9.2(c).   A sagittal T_1-weighted MRI scan in the same patient, demonstrating plaques that now appear hypointense (dark), as opposed to the hyperintense (bright) lesions revealed by the spin echo sequences.

may be reduced by using contiguous slices with a thin slice thickness. Another difficulty is distinguishing MS plaques from coarse vascular lesions (Ormerod et al., 1984) and those seen in the vasculitides, namely systemic lupus erythematosus and Behcet's disease amongst others (Miller et al., 1987). In addition, MRI cannot differentiate high intensity signals occasionally seen in healthy individuals (George et al., 1986; Hachinski et al., 1987) from MS plaques. The clinical significance of these high intensity signal lesions, also termed leukoaraiosis or unidentified bright objects (UBO) is discussed later in this chapter. Two sets of criteria pertaining to MRI lesions and strongly suggestive of multiple sclerosis have been devised, namely those of Paty et al. (1988b)(four lesions $\geqslant 3$ mm or three lesions, one of which is periventricular) and those of Fazekas et al. (1988)(three or more lesions with at least two of the following; $\geqslant 5$ mm, periventricular, infratentorial). Helpful as they are, the diagnosis of MS remains essentially a clinical one and, while MRI may facilitate the process, imaging changes cannot be regarded as pathognomonic.

MRI is a safe procedure. The recognized hazards are those which the

(a)

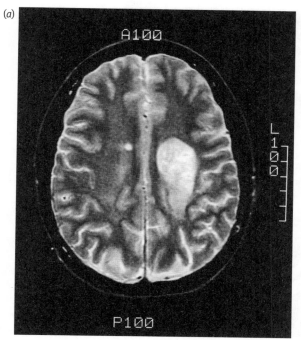

Fig. 9.3(a).   Axial T_2-weighted (spin echo) MRI, showing a large MS plaque in the left hemisphere and a smaller, circumscribed lesion in the right hemisphere.

magnetic field can exert upon ferromagnetic materials, such as certain aneurysm clips and pacemakers (New et al., 1983; Pavlicek et al., 1983). Furthermore, MRI has no measurable adverse effect on cognition (Sweetland et al., 1987). The lack of unwanted effects has made serial studies with MRI possible (Isaac et al., 1988; Miller et al., 1988; Willoughby et al., 1989). Together with the use of contrast compounds such as gadolinium-DTPA (Gd-DTPA), new light has been shed on the pathogenesis of lesion formation, for the presence of enhancement signifies a breakdown of the blood–brain barrier (BBB)(Hawkins et al., 1990) and is a consistent finding in new lesions (Miller et al., 1988; Thompson et al., 1992)(Figs. 9.3(a) and (b)). Serial studies with Gd-DTPA have also demonstrated that disruption of the BBB can precede other MRI abnormalities and clinical evidence of new lesion formation (Kermode et al., 1990a, b). In over two-thirds of patients, the duration of enhancement is less than 6 weeks (Miller et al., 1988; Thompson et al., 1992).

More recently, in an effort to increase the ability of MRI to detect acute lesions, the dose of Gd-DTPA has been trebled (i.e. 0.3 mmole/kg of Gd-DTPA), without an associated increase in side effects. In a serial study of 22 patients that first used a standard dose of GD-DTPA (0.1 mole/kg) followed 6

(b)

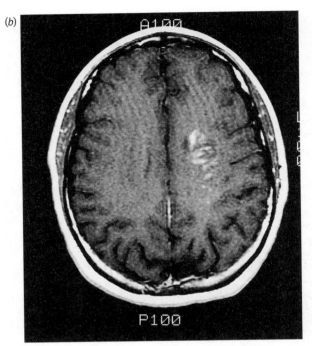

Fig. 9.3(b). Axial T_1-weighted, contrast (gadolinium-DTPA)-enhanced MRI of the same patient, showing how the large left hemisphere lesion, visible on the T_2-weighted sequence is no longer visible and has been replaced by small areas of contrast enhancement, indicative of more active disease and breakdown of the blood-brain barrier. The small right hemisphere lesion visible on the T_2-weighted scan has also disappeared on the T_1-weighted scan.

to 24 hours later with the triple dose regime, Filippi et al. (1996a) reported that the number of enhancing lesions increased from 83 (in 14 patients) to 138 (in 18 patients), namely a 28% increase and this difference was highly significant statistically ($P<0.0001$). The total lesion area per patient also increased, as did the number of large enhancing lesions, both changes proving highly significant. In a second study, Filippi et al. (1996b) replicated their results, but in a different MS population, namely those with benign MS. The particular subset of patients was chosen because their illness is charac-terized by a low frequency of clinical relapse, mild T_2-weighted lesion load, and a lower rate of disease activity as demonstrated by serial MRI with conventional Gd-DTPA dosing.

The progressive nature of brain involvement in MS is illustrated by the changes in lesion load over time. While approximately 60% of patients with clinically isolated lesions have brain abnormalities at initial presentation (Ormerod et al., 1987), this progresses to virtually 100% by the time they develop definite MS (Miller et al., 1992). Fluctuations in both lesion size and number, particularly in those with a secondary progressive type of illness have been documented (Thompson et al., 1991). The dynamic nature of the lesions plus Filippi et al.'s (1996b) finding of increased disease activity in patients whose disease was thought to be quiescent, illustrates the heterogeneity of inflammatory changes in MS and accounts for the poor correlation of neuroimaging and clinical findings reported in many studies (Jacobs et al., 1986; Isaac et al., 1988; Thompson et al., 1990). There is also MRI evidence that the amount of healthy white matter reduces with time. Stone et al. (1995) serially studied seven mildly affected relapsing–remitting MS patients with contrast-enhanced MRI at monthly intervals for durations ranging from 26 to 36 months. Although the amount of abnormal white matter signal fluctuated over the sessions (due to changes in disease activity or measurement error or both), when a mean measurement for the first 6 months was contrasted with a mean for the last 6 months, significantly less healthy white matter remained.

Relationship between MRI and cognitive abnormalities

The strength of the association between cognitive dysfunction and MRI lesion load has been influenced by the method used to quantify lesions. Two approaches have been followed: the use of rating scales to estimate the size and number of lesions or the direct quantification of lesion area/volume using computerized methods. Early studies relied on the former, which is considered inferior because it is prone to human error and produces a range of artificially restricted values (Rao, 1990).

Initial methods of direct computerized quantification relied on an approach whereby individual brain slices were displayed on a computer monitor and, using a cursor, the outline of lesions manually traced by a rater. The software calculated the total number of pixels included within the trace, which was then converted to an area (cm^2) or volume (cm^3) measurement. However, partial volume effects often made it difficult to distinguish where a lesion ended and the healthy brain began, and this lowered the inter- and intrarater reliability. More recently, with improvement in software capabilities, it has become possible for the rater to be dispensed with entirely (Wicks et al., 1992) and for the computer to segment out grey matter, white matter, cerebrospinal fluid and MS plaques (see Fig. 9.4: colour plate). This method can provide measurements of total lesion volume in the brain, plus a quantification of cortical and subcortical brain volumes. Three-dimensional reconstructed brain images allow for more precise anatomical localization of lesions and should prove of considerable benefit in the search for cerebral correlates of cognitive and emotional disorders. While undoubtedly promising, further refinement of techniques are needed. A three-way comparison between manual demarcation of lesions, a semiautomated quantification (local lesion based threshold) and intensity-based threshholding for the entire brain showed that the total lesion load measured by the first two procedures were similar, but significantly exceeded the volumes recorded by the latter (Grimaud et al., 1996).

Total lesion score and cognitive dysfunction

The majority of studies using the rating scale approach to MRI analysis have reported significant correlations between total lesion score and indices of cognitive dysfunction (Callanan et al., 1989; , Maurelli et al., 1992; Medaer et al., 1987; Anzola et al., 1990; Pozzilli et al., 1991b; Pugnetti et al., 1993; Ryan et al., 1996; Tsolaki et al., 1994; Comi et al., 1993; Franklin et al., 1988; Feinstein et al., 1992b, 1993; Ron et al., 1991).

Three studies have demonstrated that the yield of significant correlations is, however, strengthened when direct computerized quantification of total brain area is used. Rao et al. (1989a) measured total lesion area (TLA), area of the corpus callosum and ventricular brain ration (VBR), and looked for associations between these three MRI variables and 34 cognitive tests that minimized reliance on visual acuity and motor dexterity. In their analysis, age and education were controlled for. VBR was not associated with a single cognitive index, but total lesion area correlated significantly with 25, and corpus callosum atrophy with 8 cognitive measures respectively. The authors concluded that, when total lesion area exceeded a particular cut-off point (i.e. > 30 cm^2), the probability of cognitive impairment was high.

Using a similar method of lesion quantification, Feinstein et al. (1992a) investigated MRI and cognitive abnormalities in 42 patients with acute optic neuritis. Given that patients had not yet progressed to a diagnosis of MS, the lesion load in the brain was comparatively small, although lesions were detected in 55% of the sample. While significant correlations were noted between total lesion area and tests of attention, in those optic neuritis patients with a normal MRI, cognitive performance did not differ from a group of healthy controls.

Finally, Swirsky-Sacchetti et al. (1992) also noted that TLA was the best predictor of cognitive deficits, but extended their investigation by exploring regional analyses too.

Localized brain abnormalities and cognitive dysfunction

Although the MRI variable most strongly linked to various indices of cognitive dysfunction has been total lesion area (TLA), there is a lone dissenting voice. Huber et al. (1987) compared demented to non-demented MS subjects and found that atrophy of the corpus callosum and not TLA was the only distinguishing MRI variable. Other studies have also investigated the corpus callosum, and to a lesser extent the frontal lobes, searching for associations between regional MRI scores and more specific cognitive difficulties.

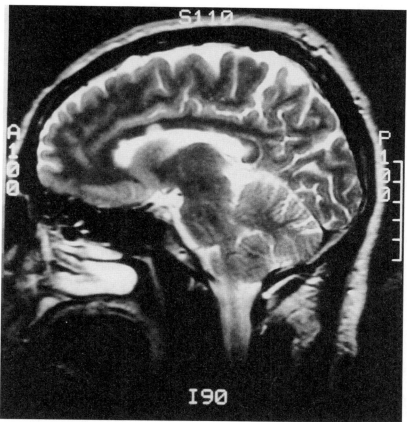

Fig. 9.5.   A mid-sagittal T_2-weighted (fast spin echo) sequence, showing the punched out appearance of lesions within the corpus callosum of a patient with MS.

Corpus callosum The corpus callosum is composed of white matter fibres linking the hemispheres and, as such, is likely to be affected by demyelination, showing signs either of atrophy and/or lesion involvement (Fig. 9.5). However, the frequency and severity with which the corpus callosum is affected in MS has not been systematically investigated, although postmortem studies suggest involvement is common and occasionally extensive (Barnard and Triggs, 1974).

The cognitive deficits most closely identified with corpus callosum abnormalities have been speed of information processing and rapid problem solving (Rao et al., 1989a). Furthermore, atrophy of the corpus callosum has also correlated significantly with deficits when verbal stimuli are presented dichotically, which may account for the difficulties experienced by some MS patients on tests of laterality and sustained attention and vigilance (Rao et al., 1989b). Poor performance on verbal fluency tasks (Controlled Oral Word

Association Task (COWAT)) has also been linked to atrophy of the anterior portion of the corpus callosum (Pozzilli et al., 1991a), an area that interconnects right and left frontal lobes. A similar observation was reported by Rao et al. (1989a), although, in this study, no attempt was made to subdivide the corpus callosum into anterior (head, genu and rostral body) and posterior (posterior callosal body, isthmus and splenium) divisions. A third MRI study associating impairment on the COWAT with left frontal pathology (Swirsky-Sacchetti et al., 1992) supports the observation that primarily frontal neural circuitry is responsible for word list generation.

Pelletier et al. (1993) used semiquantitative MRI analysis to investigate the interhemispheric transfer of auditory, sensory and motor information and noted that specific cognitive abnormalities were predominantly associated with localized areas of corpus callosum atrophy. Thus, deficits on left ear dichotic suppression were linked to atrophy of the posterior callosal region, while deficits on alternate finger tapping and cross-localization were associated with atrophy of the anterior and mid-anterior/posterior regions, respectively. Cognitive difficulties across all three modalities also correlated with the number of intrahemispheric white matter lesions which, in turn, correlated significantly with indices of corpus callosum atrophy, suggesting a complex interplay between the various anatomical and neuro-psychological variables. To explore this further, a group of patients with corpus callosum atrophy without hemispheric plaques were assessed and their performance on the cognitive tests were also found to be impaired in relation to the healthy controls. Whether these deficits could be explained on the basis of small white matter hemispheric lesions that defied macroscopic detection or some intrinsic pathological process selectively targeting the corpus callosum was, however, unclear.

Before concluding this section on the corpus callosum, some discrepant findings should be noted. Ryan et al. (1996) established that lesions in the genu were associated with abnormalities on the Benton Visual Retention Test. Why this should be is unclear, for reports of corpus callosum involvement in visuo-spatial function stress it is the posterior aspects that are implicated (Le Doux et al., 1978). Ryan et al. (1996) posit that a lesion in the genu may reflect more widespread demyelination within the corpus callosum as a whole, although their method of MRI analysis precluded exploring this possibility. Finally, sample selection may explain the failure of a MRI/PET study to report any association between pathology in the corpus callosum and cognitive deficits (Pozzilli et al., 1991b). Only patients with a relapsing–remitting disease course and mild physical disability (mean EDSS of 1.7) were included.

Frontal lobes Impairment in conceptual reasoning, perseverative responses and difficulties shifting set are consistent abnormalities reported in MS patients (Ron et al., 1991; Rao et al., 1991; McIntosh-Michaelis et al., 1991) and the test most frequently used to elicit these deficits has been the Wisconsin Card Sort Test. What is more controversial, however, is whether these abnormalities are frontal in origin and by extension, whether the WCST is predominantly a frontal lobe task (see Chapter 6).

The most robust evidence of frontal lesions and poor WCST performance comes from Arnett et al. (1994). Forty-three MS patients were divided into three groups, on the basis of their MRI findings. If lesion load was less than 20 cm^2, they were deemed cognitively intact and referred to as a control group. The remaining two groups were differentiated on the basis of their frontal lesion load into predominantly frontal or non-frontal. The performance of these groups across three subtests of the WCST (number of perseverative responses, number of categories achieved, total errors) were compared, while controlling for the effects of total lesion area and global cognitive decline. The results indicated that the 'frontal' patients performed significantly more poorly than the other groups on two WCST indices. In addition, a case report is described wherein a patient was followed up after a period of 36 months during which time his frontal lesion score increased considerably, a change accompanied by his performance on the WCST deteriorating from a baseline normal to impaired.

Swirsky-Sacchetti et al. (1992) have also reported a similar association, although their study did not control for the confounding effects of TLA, an important consideration given that TLA had earlier been shown to correlate with 'categories complete' and 'perseverative errors' on the WCST (Rao et al., 1989a). These findings beg the question, as yet unanswered, whether a predominantly non-frontal lesion load would also result in impaired performance on the WCST? Arnett et al.'s data, based on a small sample size, suggests not. However, successful performance on the WCST could depend on a number of cognitive factors, including intact attention (sustained, selective, divided), speed of information processing and working and long term memory (Arnett et al., 1994) and to suppose all these process are purely frontally mediated would be incorrect. This is supported by Foong et al. (1997), who investigated executive function in MS patients using a subset of tests from the Cambridge Neuropsychological Test Automated Battery. Correlations between test performances and frontal MRI lesion volume (ascertained via a semiautomated technique) were sought. The range of tests administered allowed the authors to dissect out different aspects of executive function and, although MS patients in general demonstrated greater impairment relative to healthy controls, within an individual some aspects were more adversely affected than others. Furthermore, poor performance on executive tasks could not be attributed solely to frontal lobe pathology as demonstrated by MRI. The study suggests 'executive function' is best viewed as an umbrella term for a number of subcomponents, which in turn are probably subserved by different, widely distributed neural systems (Burgess and Shallice, 1992). This theoretical framework helps explain the inconsistent findings pertaining to MRI studies investigating the functional relevance of frontal versus total lesion area.

Periventricular lesions There are reports of cognitive dysfunction, most frequently various aspects of memory, being associated with periventricular lesions (Reischies et al., 1988; Izquierdo et al., 1991; Pozzilli et al., 1991b; Maurelli et al., 1992), but these data are hard to interpret. Periventricular lesions are often confluent, making a more precise anatomical localisation difficult. In addition, the propensity of MS lesions for periventricular sites will generally ensure that this lesion area correlates significantly with total lesion area. The possibility of the periventricular lesions affecting the function of more distant sites, through a process of 'disconnection', or interruption of neural circuitry through demyelination, must also be considered.

In summary, MS is not the ideal disorder from which to draw specific inferences about cerebral localization of cognitive dysfunction. The advantage of MRI sensitivity in detecting lesions is frequently offset by the often widespread, large and confluent lesion pattern that makes anatomical localization, at best, imprecise.

Ventricular dilatation An initial CT report (Rao et al., 1985) of cognitive dysfunction and ventricular enlargement has largely been substantiated by the MRI data (Pozzilli et al., 1991b; Clark et al., 1992; Comi et al., 1993). The data, however, concerning third ventricular enlargement, are more equivocal, with some (Pozzilli et al., 1991b), but not others (Clark et al., 1992) reporting an association. The reasons for this may be traced to the considerable interpatient variability with respect to third ventricle size. The wide standard deviations (Clark et al., 1992) therefore, obscure a subgroup of MS patients with large third ventricles, and it is here that the most robust correlations with cognitive impairment are to be found.

Longitudinal studies

The safety of MRI has facilitated its use in longitudinal studies, where, combined with serial measures of cognitive function, it has been important in clarifying the natural history of cognitive change in MS and the brain abnormalities underlying these changes. In addition, the use of contrast-enhanced MRI has allowed the relationship between the development of acute brain lesions and their neuropsychological sequelae to be explored. The ability of longitudinal studies to record the evolution of cognitive, disease-related (e.g. physical disability, disease course, disease exacerbation) and MRI brain changes, has also shed light on the complex, and, at times, perplexing interplay between these variables.

In a follow-up study of 48 patients with clinically isolated lesions of the type seen in MS, Feinstein et al. (1992b) repeated MRI and a cognitive battery on average $4\frac{1}{2}$ years after initial assessment. Approximately half the subjects had developed MS during the follow-up period, but because of differences in MRI slice thickness between the initial and follow-up studies, direct imaging comparisons were not possible. However, indirect evidence of lesion progression was obtained by comparing cross-sectionally lesion scores in patients who had remained with clinically isolated lesions and those who had gone on to develop MS, the latter displaying a significantly higher lesion load. It was also this group who had developed a number of new cognitive deficits, prominent of which was memory impairment. A single significant correlation was reported between visual (recognition) memory and total lesion score. The presence of only one statistically significant correlation, in contrast to the multiple indices reported by other cross-sectional studies, most notably Rao et al. (1989a) was most likely due to the method of lesion detection, which relied on a rating scale as opposed to a semiautomated approach. The study was, however, important for two reasons. First, it demonstrated the progression of cognitive impairment early in the demyelination process and secondly, by controlling for a host of variables such as age, gender, education, disease duration, disease course, physical disability and emotional factors such as depression and anxiety, clearly demonstrated that it was the progression of brain pathology that determined the pace of cognitive decline.

The same conclusions were reached in 1-year (Hohol et al., 1997) and 2-year (Mariani et al., 1991) follow-up studies of patients with established MS. The Hohol study was the first MRI-cognition related investigation to use a fully automated, three-dimensional computer-assisted method of lesion quantification. Forty-four patients were assessed with MRI and the Brief Repeatable Battery of Neuropsychological Tests on admission to the study and after a duration of 1 year. In the interim they underwent MRI scanning on average every 2 weeks. Two MRI variables were obtained; total lesion volume (TLV) and brain to intracranial cavity volume ratio. At index assessment, both MRI variables correlated significantly with three of the five cognitive variables, namely 10/36 Spatial Recall Test, Symbol-Digit Modality Test and the Paced Auditory Serial Addition Task. At 1 year follow-up, cognitive decline as a group finding had not taken place. However, in the four patients who had cognitively deteriorated, total lesion volume increased more than tenfold compared to those patients whose cognitive state either improved ($n=19$) or remained constant ($n=21$). At neither index nor follow-up appointment did physical disability (EDSS) correlate with the MRI

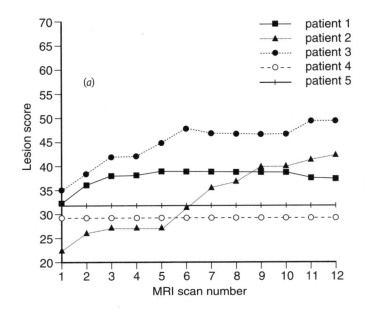

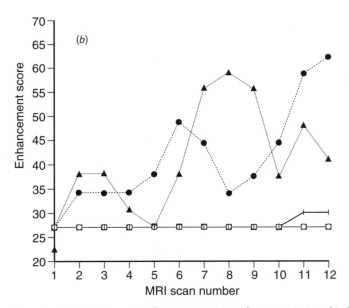

Fig. 9.6(a).   MRI lesion scores (Feinstein et al., 1993). By permission of Oxford University
Press.
(b).   Gadolinium enhancement scores (Feinstein et al., 1993). By permission of Oxford
University Press.

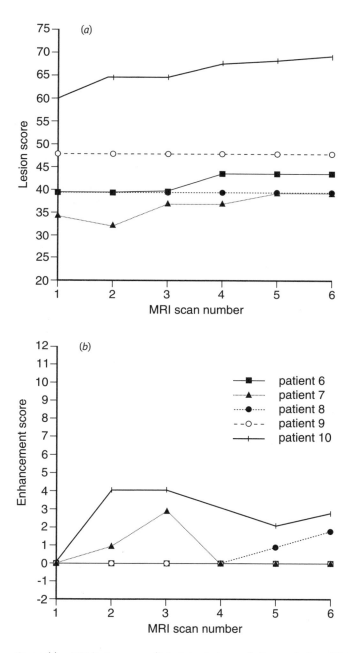

Fig. 9.7(a).   MRI lesion scores (Feinstein et al., 1993). By permission of Oxford University Press.
(b).   Gadolinium enhancement scores (Feinstein et al., 1993). By permission of Oxford University Press.

variables, confirming yet again that cognition was a more sensitive indicator than neurological signs of brain pathology.

While these studies provided evidence of change affecting brain and cognition after an interval spanning 1 to 2 years, they could not elucidate whether cognition mirrored the weekly waxing and waning in size and contrast enhancement known to occur with MS lesions. To investigate this possibility, more frequent scanning and psychometric testing were required. In a serial study over 6 months confined to patients with relapsing–remitting MS, Feinstein et al. (1993) undertook gadolinium-enhanced MRI at 2–weekly intervals in five patients with active disease (Group A) and monthly intervals in five patients with 'benign' MS (Group B). Neuropsychological testing preceeded MRI in each subject at each session. The changing total lesion scores and changing contrast-enhanced lesion scores are best viewed graphically (see Figs. 9.6(a), (b), and 9.7 (a), (b).

The study highlighted not only the variability in cognitive performance over time (see Chapter 7), but also a commensurate variability in MRI brain lesion scores. In general, tests of sensorimotor function were the most sensitive to a deteriorating brain lesion score. For other cognitive functions, practice effects exerted a powerful influence which meant patients' performances on tests such as the Stroop and PASAT continued to improve, despite a constant or even a deteriorating lesion score. Finally, the hazards of predicting what changes may occur in the brains of MS patients were clearly demonstrated. Of the five patients in Group A deemed to have active MS prior to enrolment, only two displayed longitudinal evidence of a worsening lesion score. This variability on so many fronts accounts for the failure of another gadolinium-enhanced MRI and cognitive study to report significant associations between the variables concerned (Mattioli et al., 1993).

Correlations between relaxation times and cognitive variables

The demonstration of MS plaques by MRI provides a good measure of cerebral involvement, but brain changes that are not macroscopically discernable may also be influencing cognition. T_1 and T_2 relaxation times provide just such a measure, as they reflect the presence of microscopic abnormalities such as perivascular inflammation, myelin breakdown and astrocyte hyperplasia (Allen et al., 1981). In a study that produced an association between total lesion score and only one cognitive variable, raised T_1 relaxation times in an area of normal appearing frontal white matter (see Fig. 9.8: colour plate) correlated significantly with impaired ability on tasks of abstraction, visual memory and naming (Feinstein et al., 1992b). These results have not been replicated in MS patients, although similar associations have been reported in Alzheimer's disease (Besson et al., 1990). The reluctance on the part of researchers in general to pursue studies of relaxation time abnormalities in MS (not only in relation to cognition) may be attributed to the emergence of magnetic resonance spectroscopy as a means of exploring the chemical and molecular composition of MS lesions and the surrounding, normal appearing white matter.

Magnetic Resonance Spectroscopy

Magnetic resonance spectroscopy (MRS) was first developed in the mid-1940s as a method to determine the magnetic properties of atomic nuclei. Initially used in the field of molecular physics and chemistry, it provided valuable information on molecular structure and chemical reaction rates. Biochemists have used spectroscopy to elucidate the structure of cell membranes, nucleic acids, proteins and viruses. The earliest experiments on living systems involved phosphorus (^{31}P) spectroscopy of red blood cells, excised muscle tissue and suspensions of yeast cells. This was followed by studies of systems such as whole animals, perfused organs and cellular suspensions. Other nuclei studied have included hydrogen (^{1}H), fluorine (^{19}F), carbon-13 (^{13}C), sodium (^{23}Na), potassium (^{39}K) and nitrogen (^{15}N and ^{14}N). With respect to medical research, improvements in NMR technology over the last 10–15 years have now enabled the technique to be applied to the in vivo study of the physiology and metabolism of living organisms. Of particular medical interest are in vivo proton, phosphorus and carbon spectra because the three occur in the body in compounds that play an important role in cellular metabolism and in the supply of energy. They are also present in sufficient concentrations to permit detection.

There are a number of ways in which information on biochemistry and physiology can be obtained by MR spectroscopy. One approach is to measure the levels of metabolites in diseased tissue and to compare these results with those from normal tissue. Thus, lesions such as tumours or infarcts, demonstrated via other techniques such as MRI or CT may have their chemical structure demonstrated by spectroscopy. When displaying spectra, the frequencies are not expressed in absolute units, but in relative units instead. The reason is that frequencies are not constant, but increase linearly in relation to field strength. By expressing any given frequency relative to a reference compound, the frequency value becomes constant, allowing for comparisons between measurements obtained on different systems with different field strengths. A commonly used reference compound in brain proton spectroscopy is creatine.

The application of MRS to multiple sclerosis offers new research possibilities such as evaluating a number of interesting metabolites. An example is N-acetyl aspartate (NAA), which is an amino acid found largely in neurones and therefore considered a non-specific marker of neuronal integrity. Reduction of NAA in MS is recognized as a probable measure of axonal loss in chronic lesions, whereas a partial reversal of NAA reduction may occur in acute lesions (Davie et al., 1994).

MRS can also detect mobile lipids during periods of myelin breakdown, while a rise in choline concentration (relative to creatine) may relate to changes in membrane viability in association with an inflammatory cell infiltrate. Consequently, serial MRS may play a useful role in studying the natural history of MS lesions in addition to monitoring brain changes during clinical trials (Miller, 1995).

Spectroscopy has yet to be applied to the group study of cognitive aspects of MS, although the rationale for doing so is compelling. Given the preliminary conclusions from the T_1 relaxation time data (Feinstein et al., 1992b), spectroscopy may provide more substantial evidence of neuronal destruction. There is, however, a single case report linking cognitive ability to changes noted on MRS (Rozewicz et al. 1996). A 21–year-old MS patient suffered a relapse that resulted in quadriplegia. This was associated with cognitive deficits affecting primarily left hemisphere function, i.e. the Graded Naming and Token Tests. Given her neurological deficits, a performance IQ score could not be obtained. Gadolinium-enhanced MRI done at the time revealed a number of high signal, often contrast-enhancing lesions in the white matter and cortex. Proton spectroscopy from an enhancing lesion demonstrated a decrease in the N-acetyl-aspartate (NAA)/creatine ratio, and a choline/creatine ratio that was not, initially, elevated.

The patient was treated with high dose intravenous steroids. Seven weeks after admission her EDSS had decreased from 9.0 to 6.5 and she was able to walk a few yards with assistance. Repeat neuropsychological testing and neuroimaging showed improvement on the Graded Naming and Token Test, and a marked reduction in the size of six of the lesions, with a reduction in some lesion enhancement. Repeat MRS showed a large rise in her choline/creatine ratio and a more modest increase in the NAA/creatine ratio. Increased lipid and macromolecule resonances noted in the first MRS examination had decreased at follow-up, but not to the levels found in healthy controls. Given the temporal synchronicity of cognitive, MRI and MRS changes, a more complete picture emerges of the brain changes underlying alterations in mentation.

Although informative, the case report made no mention of MRS changes in normal appearing white matter. If present, this would have supplied more subtle, widespread evidence of cerebral disorder related to cognitive dysfunction.

Leukoaraiosis

Areas of high signal intensity in the cerebral white mater may be found in healthy individuals, particularly with more advanced age, but may also

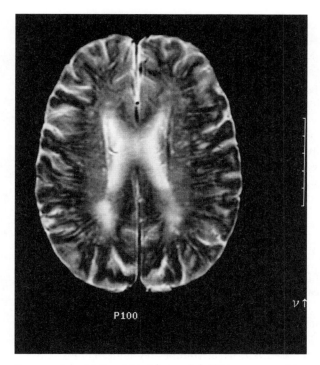

Fig. 9.9.   An axial T_2-weighted (spin echo) MRI in a 71-year-old asymptomatic, normotensive male. Note the confluent periventricular and multiple discrete, small white matter hyperintensities (leukoaraiosis) together with prominent Virchow–Robbin spaces.

accompany a host of pathological conditions such as lupus, cerebral vascular insufficiency, leukodystrophy, and bipolar affective disorder. The radiological appearance of these lesions may be indistinguishable from those seen in MS (Fig. 9.9).

Uncertainty has surrounded the pathogenesis and clinical significance of these white matter lesions in otherwise healthy subjects. With improvements in MRI imaging techniques over the past two decades, the ability to detect subtle white matter changes has increased accordingly and prompted cautionary advice from Hachinski et al. (1987) not to attribute a pathologic process to a neuroimaging sign of, as yet, unproven clinical significance. The authors put forward the term 'leukoaraiosis' derived from the Greek words 'leuko' meaning 'white', and 'araios' signifying 'loose' and implying a diminution in density. Thus, it was postulated that, for reasons which were unclear, a lessening in the density of the white matter resulted in an extravasation of fluid thinning the neural substrate and showing up as white matter high signal areas on MRI. 'Leukoaraiosis' was envisaged as a temporary term that would, in time, become obsolete as knowledge concerning pathogenesis became available. Reviewing the literature suggests that, while abandoning the term may at present be premature, some clarification has taken place.

Many of the studies have centred on elderly subjects, where the frequency of white matter hyperintensities is increased. However, in a study confined to middle-aged subjects Rao et al. (1989c) compared the neuropsychological performance of normotensive patients with ($n=10$) and without ($n=40$) MRI signs of leukoaraiosis. No cognitive differences were found between the two groups. However, the limitations of a cross-sectional approach were emphasized, and longitudinal studies advocated, before more definitive conclusions were reached. The finding of an absence of cognitive deficits is in accord with other studies involving more elderly subjects (Brant-Zawadski et al., 1985; Tupler et al., 1992).

However, a limitation of all these studies was the method of MRI assessment, which relied on a rating scale approach and was thus unable to provide estimates of total lesion area or volume. It is therefore significant that, in a study with a wide age scatter that used computerized quantification of lesion volume and functional brain imaging (PET), significant cognitive and other radiological differences were found between patients with varying degrees of white matter lesions (DeCarli et al., 1995). The crucial point relates to threshold. A white matter hyperintensity volume in excess of 0.5% (10 cm^2) of intracranial volume was associated not only with cognitive impairment, but also with increased ventricular volume and reduced brain volume. Exploring the role of each of these imaging variables in cognitive performance, a regression analysis highlighted that the white matter lesions were an independent predictor of cognitive dysfunction. In addition, if white matter lesion volume exceeded the threshold, frontal lobe metabolism was decreased in association with impaired neuropsychological performance on frontally mediated tasks. Despite all adults being deemed healthy prior to enrolment, a significant association emerged between increased white matter lesions and raised systolic blood pressure.

DeCarli and colleagues provide sound evidence linking white matter changes in clinically healthy adults to mild, subclinical degrees of hypertension, cognitive impairment and brain atrophy. As these changes are all more common with increasing age, the study offers the most complete explanation yet of why white matter high signal lesions are so frequently reported in the elderly. The notion of lesions having to exceed a particular threshold of white matter volume before cognitive problems manifest harkens back to the finding in MS patients linking a total lesion area exceeding 20 cm^2 to cognitive dysfunction (Rao et al., 1989a). Notwithstanding this result, there remains a subset of younger, healthy patients, albeit small in number, with white matter lesions of uncertain etiology. Longitudinal studies involving these subjects would prove informative.

Positron emission tomography (PET) and single photon emission computerized tomography (SPECT)

The often widespread and confluent nature of MS lesions that may disconnect neural networks at multiple points, and to varying degrees, has made MS a particularly problematic disorder for PET and SPECT studies. The role of functional imaging in MS has therefore largely been to demonstrate evidence of widespread cerebral blood flow and metabolic abnormalities, and this it has successfully achieved. Given this fact, the positive association between global estimates of cognitive impairment and cerebral involvement becomes easier to understand.

In the most comprehensive of three published studies, Brooks et al. (1984) compared 15 MS patients in remission to 13 normal controls, looking at regional cerebral utilization, oxygen extraction, cerebral blood flow and blood volume. A significant global reduction in cerebral oxygen utilisation and blood flow were found both in the white and grey matter of the MS patients. These deficits were associated with cortical atrophy on CT and with evidence of intellectual decline as assessed by the Wechsler Adult Intelligence Scale. No regional abnormalities were found, and the authors failed to note a correlation between the functional abnormalities displayed on PET and either disease duration or severity.

Herscovitch et al. (1984), in a single case report of a 24-year-old patient with aphasia, apraxia and left-sided hemiparesis with sensory changes, demonstrated a lesion in the right cerebral white matter on CT, while PET showed a reduction in regional cerebral blood flow (rCBF) in the frontoparietal cortex superficial to the lesion. Subsequent improvement in rCBF was associated with clinical remission. Although the association between the structural and functional abnormalities would have been improved by MRI as opposed to CT, to date no such study has been undertaken.

In the only published SPECT report, Pozzilli et al. (1991b) scanned 17 MS patients and 17 matched, healthy controls using 99m (99mTc) hexamethylpropyleneamine oxime (HMPAO) SPECT. A ratio of regional to whole brain activity, measured by SPECT, demonstrated a significant reduction in the frontal lobes and left temporal lobe of the patient sample. Deficits in verbal memory and verbal fluency correlated with the reduction in left temporal lobe 99mTc-HMPAO uptake.

There is also a single small PET study that reported the results of a cognitive activation paradigm. Scheremata et al. (1984) used a word learning activation task in a case control study involving three MS subjects and three healthy matched controls. They found reduced metabolism in both temporal, and to a lesser extent, frontal lobes of the MS patients. Although information was not present for all brain areas, the authors concluded that their results were indicative of generalized cortical hypometabolism.

Summary

- MRI is considerably more sensitive that CT in detecting MS plaques in the brain. Plaques are typically periventricular in distribution.
- MRI may also demonstrate abnormalities of the corpus callosum (atrophy or the presence of lesions) and generalized cerebral atrophy.
- The lesions demonstrated by MRI are not pathognomonic for MS, and a host of neurological disorders, e.g. vascular changes, HIV dementia, metachromatic leukodystrophy, to name but a few, may give rise to an indistinguishable picture.
- The use of contrast (gadolinium-DTPA) -enhanced MRI may demonstrate the presence of acute MS lesions, with enhancement indicative of breakdown in the blood–brain barrier.
- MRI is a safe procedure and therefore ideally suited to longitudinal studies requiring repeated scans.
- Total lesion area and volume are significantly associated with many indices of cognitive dysfunction.
- Atrophy and/or lesions of the corpus callosum are present in patients with delayed speed of information processing and difficulties transferring information between the cerebral hemispheres.
- Serial MRI and cognitive studies have shown that psychomotor tasks are the most sensitive indicators of a deteriorating brain lesion load. However, patients may retain the ability to benefit from practice and improve their psychometric performances on tests such as those of speed of information processing, despite a worsening in their brain MRI picture.
- Abnormal T_1 relaxation times in normal appearing white matter have also been found to correlate with cognitive abnormalities.
- NMR spectroscopy provides in vivo concentrations of important metabolites such as N-acetyl aspartate and choline, which although non-specific, become abnormal to various degrees in MS, depending on the severity and stage of lesion formation and resolution. Changes in their concentrations may correlate with cognitive decline and improvement. Spectroscopy thus adds to what is known about MS lesions from MRI.
- Functional neuroimaging (PET and SPECT) is not particularly well suited to MS, because the often widespread and confluent lesions interrupt or diminish cerebral blood flow (or metabolism) at multiple points, making data interpretation difficult. As such, only a handful of cognition related studies have been completed, all but one with poor sample size.

References

Allen IV, Glover G, Andersen R. (1981) Abnormalities in the macroscopically normal white matter in cases of mild or spinal multiple sclerosis. *Acta Neuropathologica (Berlin)*, Suppl., **7**, 176–8.

Andrew EE, Bydder G, Griffiths J, Iles R, Styles P. (1990) *Clinical Magnetic Resonance Imaging and Spectroscopy*. Chichester: John Wiley.

Anzola GP, Bevilacqua L, Cappa SF et al. (1990) Neuropsychological assessment in patients with relapsing–remitting multiple sclerosis and mild functional impairment: correlation with magnetic resonance imaging. *Journal of Neurology, Neurosurgery and Psychiatry*, **53**, 142–5.

Arnett PA, Rao SM, Bernardin L, Grafman J, Yetkin FZ, Lobeck L. (1994) Relationship between frontal lobe lesions and Wisconsin Card Sort Test performance in patients with multiple sclerosis. *Neurology*, **44**, 420–5.

Barnard RO, Triggs M. (1974) Corpus callosum and multiple sclerosis. *Journal of Neurology, Neurosurgery and Psychiatry*, **37**, 1259–64.

Besson JAO, Crawford JR, Parker DM et al. (1990) Multimodal imaging in Alzheimer's disease. The relationship between MRI, SPECT, cognitive and pathological changes. *British Journal of Psychiatry*, **157**, 216–20.

Brandt-Zawadski M, Fein G, Van Dyke C, Kiernan R, Davenport L, de Groot J. (1985) MR imaging of the aging brain: patchy white matter lesions and dementia. *American Journal of Neuroradiology*, **6**, 675–82.

Brooks DJ, Leenders KL, Head G, Marshall J, Legg NJ, Jones T. (1984) Studies on regional cerebral oxygen utilisation and cognitive function in multiple sclerosis. *Journal of Neurology, Neurosurgery and Psychiatry*, **47**, 1182–91.

Burgess PW, Shallice T. (1992) Fractionation of the frontal lobe syndrome. *Revue of Neuropsychology*, **3**, 345–70.

Callanan MM, Logsdail SJ, Ron MA, Warrington EK. (1989) Cognitive impairment in patients with clinically isolated lesions of the type seen in multiple sclerosis. *Brain*, **112**, 361–74.

Clark CM, James G, Li D, Oger J, Paty D, Klonoff H. (1992) Ventricular size, cognitive function and depression in patients with multiple sclerosis. *The Canadian Journal of Neurological Sciences*, **19**, 352–6.

Comi G, Filippi M, Martinelli V et al. (1993) Brain magnetic resonance imaging correlates of cognitive impairment in multiple sclerosis. *Journal of Neurological Sciences*, **115** (Suppl.), 66–73.

Davie CA, Hawkins CP, Barker GJ et al. (1994) Serial proton magnetic resonance spectroscopy in acute multiple sclerosis lesions. *Brain*, **117**, 49–58.

DeCarli C, Murphy DGM, Tranh M et al. (1995) The effect of white matter hyperintensity volume on brain structure, cognitive performance and cerebral metabolism of glucose in 51 healthy adults. *Neurology*, **45**, 2077–84.

Fazekas F, Offenbacher H, Fuchs S et al. (1988) Criteria for an increased specificity of MRI interpretation in elderly subjects with suspected multiple sclerosis. *Neurology*, **38**, 1822–5.

Feinstein A, Youl B, Ron MA. (1992a) Acute optic neuritis. A cognitive and magnetic resonance imaging study. *Brain*, **115**, 1403–15.

Feinstein A, Kartsounis LD, Miller DH, Youl BD, Ron MA. (1992b) Clinically isolated lesions of the type seen in multiple sclerosis: a cognitive, psychiatric and MRI follow-up study. *Journal of Neurology, Neurosurgery and Psychiatry*, **55**, 869–76.

Feinstein A, Ron MA, Thompson A. (1993) A serial study of psychometric and magnetic resonance imaging changes in multiple sclerosis. *Brain*, **116**, 569–602.

Filippi M, Yousry T, Campi A et al. (1996a) Comparison of triple dose versus standard dose gadolinium-DTPA for detection of MRI enhancing lesions in patients with MS. *Neurology*, **46**, 379–84.

Filippi M, Capra R, Campi A et al. (1996b) Triple dose of gadolinium-DTPA and delayed MRI in patients with benign multiple sclerosis. *Journal of Neurology, Neurosurgery and Psychiatry*, **60**, 526–30.

Foong J, Rozewicz L, Quaghebeur G et al. (1997) Executive function in multiple sclerosis. The role of frontal lobe pathology. *Brain*, **120**, 15–26.

Franklin GM, Heaton RK, Nelson LM, Filley CM, Seibert C. (1988) Correlation of neuropsychological and MRI findings in chronic–progressive multiple sclerosis. *Neurology*, **38**, 1826–9.

George AE, de Leon MJ, Kalnin A, Rosner L, Goodgold A, Chase N. (1986) Leukoencephalopathy in normal and pathological aging: 2. MRI of brain lucencies. *American Journal of Neuroradiology*, **7**, 567–70.

Glydensted C. (1976) Computer tomography of the cerebrum in multiple sclerosis. *Neuroradiology*, **12**, 33–42.

Grimaud J, Lai M, Thorpe J et al. (1996) Quantification of MRI lesion load in multiple sclerosis: a comparison of three computer-assisted techniques. *Magenetic Resonance Imaging*, **14**, 494–505.

Hachinski VC, Potter P, Merskey H. (1987) Leuko-araiosis. *Archives of Neurology*, **44**, 21–3.

Hawkins CP, Munro PMG, Mackenzie F et al. (1990) Duration and selectivity of blood–brain barrier breakdown in chronic relapsing experimental allergic encephalomyelitis studied by gadolinium-DTPA and protein markers. *Brain*, **113**, 365–78.

Herscovitch P, Trotter JL, Lemann W, Raichle ME. (1984) Positron emission tomography (PET) in active MS: demonstration of demyelination and diaschisis. *Neurology*, **34** (suppl 1), 78.

Hohol MJ, Guttmann CRG, Orav J et al. (1997) Serial neuropsychological assessment and magnetic resonance imaging analysis in multiple sclerosis. *Archives of Neurology*, **54**, 1018–25.

Huber SJ, Paulsen GW, Shuttleworth EC et al. (1987) Magnetic resonance imaging correlates of dementia in multiple sclerosis. *Archives of Neurology*, **44**, 732–6.

Isaac C, Li DKB, Genton M et al. (1988) Multiple sclerosis: a serial study using MRI in relapsing patients. *Neurology*, **38**, 1511–15.

Izquierdo G, Campoy Jr F, Mir J, Gonzalez M, Martinez-Parra C. (1991) Memory and learning disturbances in multiple sclerosis. MRI lesions and neuropsychological correlation. *European Journal of Radiology*, **13**, 220–4.

Jacobs L, Kinkel WR, Polachini I, Kinkel P. (1986) Correlations of nuclear magnetic resonance imaging, computerised tomography and clinical profiles in multiple sclerosis. *Neurology*, **36**, 27–34.

Kermode AG, Thompson AJ, Tofts P et al. (1990a) Breakdown of the blood–brain barrier precedes symptoms and other MRI signs of new lesions in multiple sclerosis.

Brain, **113**, 1477–89.

Kermode AG, Tofts PS. Thompson AJ et al. (1990b) Heterogeneity of blood–brain barrier changes in multiple sclerosis: an MRI study with gadolinium-DTPA enhancement. *Neurology*, **40**, 229–35.

Kurtzke JF. (1983) Rating neurologic impairment in multiple sclerosis: an expanded disability scale. *Neurology*, **33**, 1444–52.

Le Doux JE, Wilson DH, Gazzaniga MS. (1978) Block design performance following callosal sectioning. *Archives of Neurology*, **35**, 506–8.

Mariani C, Farina E, Cappa SF et al. (1991). Neuropsychological assessment in multiple sclerosis: a follow-up study with magnetic resonance imaging. *Journal of Neurology*, **238**, 395–400.

Mattioli F, Cappa SF, Cominelli C et al. (1993) Serial study of neuropsychological performance and gadolinium-enhanced MRI in MS. *Acta Neurologica Scandinavica*, **87**, 465–8.

Maurelli M, Marchioni E, Cerretano R et al. (1992) Neuropsychological assessment in MS: clinical, neurophysiological and neuroradiological relationships. *Acta Neurologica Scandinavica*, **86**, 124–8.

Medaer R, Nelissen E, Appel B, Swert M, Geutjens J, Callaert H. (1987) Magnetic resonance imaging and cognitive functioning in multiple sclerosis. *Journal of Neurology*, **235**, 86–9.

McIntosh-Michaelis SA, Roberts MH, Wilkinson SM, Diamond ID, McLellan DL, Martin JP, Spackman AJ. (1991) The prevalence of cognitive impairment in a community sample of multiple sclerosis. *British Journal of Clinical Psychology*, **30**, 333–48.

Miller DH. (1995) Magnetic resonance imaging and spectroscopy in multiple sclerosis. *Current Opinion in Neurology*, **8**, 210–15.

Miller DH, Johnson G, Tofts PS, MacManus D, McDonald WI. (1989) Precise relaxation time measurements of normal appearing white matter in inflammatory central nervous system disease. *Magnetic Resonance Imaging in Medicine*, **11**, 331–6.

Miller DH, Morrissey SP, McDonald WI. (1992) The prognostic significance of brain MRI at presentation with a single clinical episode of suspected demyelination. A 5 year follow-up study. *Neurology*, (suppl. 3), 427.

Miller DH, Ormerod IEC, Gibson A, du Boulay EPGH, Rudge P, McDonald WI. (1987) MR brain scanning in patients with vasculitis: differentiation from MS. *Neuroradiology*, **29**, 226–31.

Miller DH, Rudge P, Johnson G et al. (1988) Serial gadolinium enhanced MRI in multiple sclerosis. *Brain*, **111**, 927–39.

New PFJ, Rosen BR, Brady TJ et al. (1983) Potential hazards and artifacts of ferromagnetic and non-ferromagnetic surgical and dental material and devices in nuclear magnetic resonance imaging. *Radiology*, **147**, 139–48.

Ormerod IEC, Johnson G, MacManus D, du Boulay EPHG, McDonald WI. (1986) Relaxation times of apparently normal cerebral white matter in multiple sclerosis. *Acta Radiologica* (Suppl.), **369**, 496.

Ormerod IEC, Miller DH, McDonald WI et al. (1987) The role of NMR imaging in the assessment of multiple sclerosis and isolated neurological lesions. *Brain*, **110**, 1579–616.

Ormerod IEC, Roberts RC, du Boulay EPGH. (1984) NMR in multiple sclerosis and cerebral vascular disease. *Lancet*, **ii**, 1334–5.

Paty DW, Hashimoto SA, Hooge J et al. (1988a) Magnetic resonance imaging (MRI) in multiple sclerosis: a prospective evaluation of usefulness in diagnosis. *Neurology*, **38**, 180–5.

Paty DW, Oger JJ, Kastrukoff LF et al. (1988b) MRI in the diagnosis of MS: a prospective study with comparison of clinical evaluation, evoked potentials, oligoclonal banding, and CT. *Neurology*, **38**, 180–5.

Pavlicek W, Geisinger M, Castle L et al. (1983) The effects of nuclear magnetic resonance imaging on patients with cardiac pacemakers. *Radiology*, **147**, 149–53.

Pelletier J, Habib M, Lyon-Caen O, Salamon G, Poncet M, Khalil R. (1993) Functional and magnetic resonance imaging correlates of callosal involvement in multiple sclerosis. *Archives of Neurology*, **50**, 1077–82.

Pozzilli C, Bastianello S, Padovani A et al. (1991a) Anterior corpus callosum atrophy and verbal fluency in multiple sclerosis. *Cortex*, **27**, 441–5.

Pozzilli C, Passafiumi D, Bernardi S et al. (1991b) SPECT, MRI and cognitive functions in multiple sclerosis. *Journal of Neurology, Neurosurgery and Psychiatry*, **54**, 110–15.

Pugnetti L, Mendozzi L, Motta A et al. (1993) MRI and cognitive patterns in relapsing–remitting multiple sclerosis. *Journal of the Neurological Sciences*, 115 (suppl) 59–65.

Rabins PV, Brooks BR, O' Donnell P et al. (1986) Structural brain correlates of emotional disorder in multiple sclerosis. *Brain*, **109**, 585–97.

Rao SM. (1990) Neuroimaging correlates of cognitive dysfunction. In *Neurobehavioural Aspects of Multiple Sclerosis*, ed. SM Rao. pp 118–35. New York: Oxford University Press.

Rao SM, Bernardin L, Ellington L, Ryan SB, Burg LS. (1989b) Cerebral disconnection in multiple sclerosis. Relationship to atrophy of the corpus callosum. *Archives of Neurology*, **46**, 918–20.

Rao SM, Glatt S, Hammeke TA et al. (1985) Chronic–progressive multiple sclerosis: relationship between cerebral ventricular size and neuropsychological impairment. *Archives of Neurology*, **42**, 678–82.

Rao SM, Leo GJ, Bernardin L, Unverzagt F. (1991) Cognitive dysfunction in multiple sclerosis. 1. Frequency, patterns and prediction. *Neurology*, **41**, 6685–91.

Rao SM, Leo GJ, Haughton VM, St. Aubin-Faubert P, Bernardin L. (1989a) Correlation of magnetic resonance imaging with neuropsychological testing in multiple sclerosis. *Neurology*, **39**, 161–6.

Rao SM, Mittenberg W, Bernardin L, Haughton V, Leo GJ. (1989c) Neuropsychological test findings in subjects with leukoaraiosis. *Archives of Neurology*, **46**, 40–4.

Reischies FM, Baum K, Brau H, Hedde JP, Schwindt G. (1988) Cerebral magnetic resonance imaging findings in multiple sclerosis. Relation to disturbance of affect, drive and cognition. *Archives of Neurology*, **45**, 1114–16.

Ron MA, Callanan MM, Warrington EK. (1991) Cognitive abnormalities in multiple sclerosis: a psychometric and MRI study. *Psychological Medicine*, **21**, 59–68.

Rozewicz L, Langdon DW, Davie CA, Thompson AJ, Ron MA. (1996) Resolution of left hemisphere cognitive dysfunction in multiple sclerosis with magnetic resonance correlates: a case report. *Cognitive Neuropsychiatry*, **1**, 17–25.

Ryan L, Clark CM, Klonoff H, Li D, Paty D. (1996) Patterns of cognitive impairment in relapsing-remitting multiple sclerosis and their relationship to neuropathology on magnetic resonance images. *Neuropsychology*, **10**, 176–93.

Scheremata WA, Seush S, Knight D, Ziajka P. (1984) Altered cerebral metabolism in multiple sclerosis. *Neurology*, **34** (suppl 1), 118.

Spiegel SM, Vinuela F, Fox AJ, Pelz DM. (1985) CT of multiple sclerosis. Reassessment of delayed scanning with high doses of contrast material. *American Journal of Roentgenology*, **145**, 497–500.

Stone LA, Albert PS, Smith ME et al. (1995) Changes in the amount of diseased white matter over time in patients with relapsing–remitting multiple sclerosis. *Neurology*, **45**, 1808–14.

Sweetland J, Kertesz A, Prato FS, Nantau K. (1987) The effect of magnetic resonance imaging in human cognition. *Magnetic Resonance Imaging*, **5**, 129–35.

Swirsky-Sacchetti T, Mitchell DR, Seward J et al. (1992) Neuropsychological and structural brain lesions in multiple sclerosis. a regional analysis. *Neurology*, **42**, 1291–5.

Thompson AJ, Kermode AG, MacManus DG et al. (1990) Patterns of disease activity in multiple sclerosis: clinical and magnetic resonance imaging study. *British Medical Journal*, **300**, 631–4.

Thompson AJ, Kermode AG, Wicks D et al. (1991) Major differences in the dynamics of primary and secondary progressive multiple sclerosis. *Annals of Neurology*, **29**, 53–62.

Thompson AJ, Miller D, Youl B et al. (1992) Serial gadolinium enhanced MRI in relapsing remitting multiple sclerosis of varying disease duration. *Neurology*, **42**, 60–3.

Tsolaki M, Drevelegas A, Karachristianou S, Kapinas K, Divanoglou D, Routsonis K. (1994) Correlation of dementia, neuropsychological and MRI findings in multiple sclerosis. *Dementia*, **5**, 48–52.

Tupler LA, Coffey CE, Logue PE, Djang WT, Fagan SM. (1992) Neuropsychological importance of subcortical white matter hyperintensity. *Archives of Neurology*, **49**, 1248–52.

Warren KG, Ball MJ, Paty DW, Banna M (1976) Computer tomography in disseminated sclerosis. *Canadian Journal of Neurological Science*, **3**, 211–16.

Wicks DAG, Tofts PS, Miller DH et al. (1992) Volume measurement of multiple sclerosis lesions with magnetic resonance images. *Neuroradiology*, **34**, 475–9.

Willoughby EW, Grochowski E, Li DKB, Oger J, Kastrukoff LF, Paty DW (1989) Serial magnetic resonance scanning in multiple sclerosis: a second prospective study in relapsing patients. *Annals of Neurology*, **25**, 43–9.

Young SW. (1984) *Nuclear Magnetic Resonance Imaging: Basic Principles*. New York: Raven Press.

Young IR, Hall AS, Pallis CA, Bydder GM, Legg NJ, Steiner RE. (1981) Nuclear magnetic resonance imaging of the brain in multiple sclerosis. *Lancet*, **ii**, 1063–6.

10

Multiple sclerosis: a subcortical, white matter dementia?

Medical taxonomy is subject to periodic revision, an inevitable consequence of new information derived from increasingly sophisticated clinical and laboratory investigations. The classification of dementia illustrates this very well. For the greater part of this century, the term dementia was considered synonymous with cortical pathology, of which Alzheimer's disease was the most frequent and well described example. To be sure, Kinnear Wilson had, in 1912, described a distinctive pattern of neurobehavioural disturbance secondary to basal ganglia pathology, but his ideas were not developed in any systematic way for over 60 years. Since 1974, the concept of a different form of dementia primarily affecting subcortical structures and with a distinct clinical profile has gained wide acceptance in psychiatry, neurology and neuropsychology. While there have been those querying the validity of a 'subcortical dementia' syndrome (Hakim and Mathieson, 1979; Whitehouse et al., 1982), these doubts have largely been submerged under the weight of opinion supporting the concept.

The fourth edition of the *Diagnostic and Statistical Manual of the American Psychiatric Association (DSM-1V)*(APA, 1994) has not created a specific category of 'subcortical dementia', but has, instead, approached the issue of the classification of dementia in a more piecemeal fashion, by listing specific causes, many of which are essentially subcortical pathological processes, i.e. HIV infection, Parkinson's and Huntington's disease and multiple sclerosis. Dementia according to the DSM-1V requires the presence of four main characteristics: memory loss; one (or more) features of impaired cognition listed as aphasia, agnosia, apraxia and impaired executive function; the cognitive deficits must lead to significant impairment in occupational or social functioning and represent a significant decline from premorbid levels of functioning and finally, the cognitive disturbance cannot be solely accounted for by a delirium. These basic tenets are regarded as essential prerequisites for the diagnosis, although when it comes to specific causes of dementia, for example, Huntington's disease, descriptive details regarded as characteristic of the disorder are added to the four cardinal requirements. Inherent in this approach is a recognition that different causes of dementia are associated with their own particular constellation of signs and symptoms, but the DSM-1V manual stops short of officially endorsing a cortical–subcortical neurobehavioural divide.

This reticence is understandable, for important questions remain to be answered. This chapter will review the evidence, clinical, anatomical, and physiological that underlies the concept of a subcortical dementia. As the term is a broad rubric encompassing different anatomical areas, the focus will be restricted to pathology predominantly affecting the cerebral white matter and whether this is associated with a recognizable neurobehavioural syndrome. Reference will be made to multiple sclerosis and other white matter diseases and similarities sought in their effects on mentation. These features will be contrasted with those derived from the cortical and subcortical grey matter dementias.

Subcortical dementia

Although Wilson (1912) had noted that patients with hepatolenticular degeneration showed an absence of agnosia, apraxia and less severe memory impairment compared to patients with senile dementia, it is Albert et al. (1974) who are generally acknowledged as first giving impetus to the concept of subcortical dementia. In their report of five cases of supranuclear palsy and their literature review of a further 42 cases, four characteristic features were described, namely forgetfulness, a slowness of though processes, emotional or personality changes (summarized as apathy or depression interspersed with irritability), and an impaired ability to manipulate acquired knowledge. The latter referred to difficulties with calculation or abstraction. The absence of aphasia, agnosia and apraxia was again evident. Albert and colleagues were struck by the similarities in clinical presentation between patients with subcortical dementia and those with dementia secondary to bilateral frontal lobe pathology, and noted that patients in both groups may also display signs of pseudobulbar palsy including a pseudobulbar affect, i.e. forced laughing or crying. This overlap was considered a natural consequence of the extensive neural connections linking subcortical structures to the frontal cortex, a theme that will be expanded on later in this chapter.

McHugh and Folstein (1975) added to the emergent concept by demonstrating that patients with Huntington's disease showed many of the same behavioural characteristics as those with PSP, which, in turn, were distinct from those with Alzheimer's disease and the Wernicke–Korsakoff syndrome. The cortical–subcortical dichotomy was further validated in time by the results from studies of patients with pathology in the substantia nigra and thalamus. The emphasis in these early studies was, however, focused almost exclusively on disorders affecting the deep grey matter. Thus, a decade after Albert et al.'s (1974) landmark paper, Cummings (1986), in reviewing a burgeoning literature took Huntington's and Parkinson's disease as the prototypical subcortical conditions against which the findings from cortical dementias, predominantly Alzheimer's disease, were compared.

Neuropsychological features

A cardinal feature of the subcortical dementias is a reduction in cognitive speed, or a slowness in information processing, also termed bradyphrenia. This occurs in excess of any motor difficulties. Patients with cortical dementias are largely spared these difficulties. While both groups suffer from memory impairment, the subcortical patients successfully encode new information, but have trouble retrieving it, whereas the patients with predominantly cortical involvement struggle with encoding and are not aided by cues or recognition prompts. Language, apart from dysarthria and mild anomia, is usually not affected in the subcortical dementias, which contrasts with the expressive and non-expressive difficulties experienced by patients with predominantly cortical involvement. Different aspects of visuospatial and abstracting difficulties are present in both groups. Cortical involvement is more likely to lead to poor copying skills, while subcortical involvement is associated with problems manipulating egocentric space (e.g. map reading). Deficits in abstracting and categorization generally appear earlier and with greater severity in the cortical dementias. Attention and vigilance may be affected in both groups.

Psychiatric features

The cortical–subcortical division is harder to sustain if based on psychiatric as opposed to cognitive discriminators. This reflects the more diffuse nature of psychiatric symptomatology, in general, and explains why particular syndromes and symptoms have defied easy localization. There are many reports of depression, personality change, mania and psychosis occurring in subcortical conditions, but the same may be applied to dementias that are cortical in origin, and it would be incorrect to suggest that one group is predominantly affected. An additional problem is how one defines the various terms. Thus depression may refer to a transient symptom or an enduring, disabling syndrome and equating the two, or a failure to distinguish how studies have dealt with this question, will lead to comparisons that lack validity. Similarly, psychosis is a broad term that, depending on definition, may refer to delusions, hallucinations, thought disorder, catatonia or various combinations of these symptoms. How one defines psychosis has been subject to periodic revision and the criteria for including or excluding psychotic patients from studies has generally been arbitrary, e.g. the distinction made between psychotic patients with or without delirium or dementia. While there are strong data demonstrating that psychosis is a frequent concomitant of subcortical conditions such as Huntington's disease (Dewhurst et al., 1969; Caine and Shoulson, 1983), an equally firm association has linked the most common and disabling of all psychotic illnesses, namely schizophrenia to predominantly cortical involvement (Suddath et al., 1990; Harvey et al., 1993). Attempts at qualitatively differentiating subcortical from cortical based psychotic features have met with mixed results. Neither Davison and Bagley (1969) nor Feinstein and Ron (1990) noted differences, although Cummings (1986) reported that patients with Alzheimer's disease generally had more severe dementia and delusions with a simpler content than patients with subcortical dementias, whose intellectual impairment was less and whose delusional thought content was consequently more complex.

Summarizing the cognitive and psychiatric findings with respect to subcortical dementia, there is firmer evidence of a discrete cognitive as opposed to a psychiatric profile. However, 'subcortical dementia' refers to a syndrome encompassing both cognitive and emotional/behavioural changes, and a closer inspection of the relevant neuroanatomy and neurophysiology explains why a degree of overlap with the cortical dementias is inevitable.

Subcortical neuroanatomy

Frontal–subcortical circuits and behaviour

There is a rich network of bidirectional white matter tracts that connect the frontal lobes to other areas of the brain. While there is no lobe that does not have frontal connections, of particular interest are those frontal subcortical circuits that are known to subserve discrete behavioural syndromes. Five frontal–subcortical circuits have been demonstrated (Alexander et al., 1986; Alexander and Crutcher, 1990) and their neuroanatomy and functional characteristics summarized (Cummings, 1993). All begin in the frontal lobes, project to the striatum (caudate, putamen, and ventral striatum) and thereafter to the globus pallidus and substantia nigra, from where they relay with specific thalamic nuclei before completing the circuit by returning to the frontal area of origin. Although this overall pattern of connections is followed by all five circuits, each circuit is discrete and within each anatomical area will relay with circuit specific nuclei. Of the five circuits, three originate in separate prefrontal cortical areas, namely dorsolateral prefrontal (DLPF) cortex, lateral orbital cortex and anterior cingulate cortex. The remaining two circuits begin in the supplementary motor area and frontal eye fields, respectively. The three prefrontal circuits have subsidiary pathways at various stages throughout their course and send and receive connections to, and from, related limbic structures. As the circuit progresses from cortex to subcortex, so the neurones funnel into increasingly smaller areas, all the while maintaining their parallel and distinct anatomical integrity. This 'squeezing' of the circuits helps explain how lesions situated at various points along the pathways give rise to differing clinical presentations.

Each prefrontal circuit is associated with a specific behavioural syndrome. Lesions located in the DLPF cortex produce deficits with executive function, namely planning, organizing, sequencing and abstracting. Lesions in the lateral orbitofrontal area produce a syndrome characterized by changes in personality, typically of the labile, disinhibited, impulsive and aggressive type. Patients may appear irritable, euphoric, overtalkative and display a lack of social tact. They differ from individuals with DLPF pathology, by performing normally on tests that challenge executive function. Anterior cingulate pathology typically produces abnormalities of motivation and individuals may present as profoundly apathetic or abulic.

Lesions affecting the striatal structures may produce clinical states similar to those described above, depending on the extent to which the pathological process remains localized. This becomes increasingly less likely as the circuit projects posteroinferiorly so that lesions affecting the globus pallidus or thalamus do not produce a discrete syndrome, but rather a mixture of signs and symptoms. Thus, the clinical picture may be a combination of disinhibition and irritability (orbitofrontal syndrome), reduced motivation and interest (medial frontal–anterior cingulate syndrome) and neuropsychological deficits (DLPF syndrome). These circuits subserve not only personality attributes, but mood as well. While mania and obsessive compulsive behaviour have been linked to dysfunction of the orbitofrontal circuits, depression may arise from lesions affecting the orbitofrontal or DLPF circuits.

Cerebral white matter

Separating the cerebral cortices from the ventricular system, the cerebral white matter comprises three main types of fibres. The projection fibres reciprocally link the cortex to more distant structures such as the brain stem, association fibres connect regions in the same hemisphere and commissural fibres link the two hemispheres. This widespread neural network subserves many functions ranging from maintaining alertness (the reticular activating system) to facilitating more complex aspects such as mood and memory. The major neurotransmitter systems (noradrenaline from the locus ceruleus, serotonin from the raphe nuclei, dopamine from the tegmentum, acetylcholine from the nucleus basalis of Meynert) are dependent on the integrity of the white matter, chiefly the medial forebrain bundle as they traverse from brainstem and midbrain to the cortex. Release of neurotransmitters is, however, dependent on axonal conduction and the latter is, in turn, dependent on myelin. Thus, in demyelinating disorders such as multiple sclerosis, impaired neural conduction may vary from slowing to a complete interruption of transmission. It is, however, unclear whether in vivo evidence of altered neurotransmitter metabolism in a white matter disease such as MS (Johansson and Roos, 1974; Markianos and Sfagos, 1988) is directly attributable to demyelination or an epiphenomenon (i.e. secondary to mood change, a response to stress).

Pathogenesis of subcortical dementia

One conceptual distinction has been to regard cortical functions as *instrumental* and subcortical as *fundamental* (Albert, 1978). Instrumental functions refer to discrete aspects of cognition such as language, reading, calculation, memory, and praxis, which are all primarily dependent on neocortical areas. Fundamental functions include less highly evolved activities such as attention, arousal, motivation and mood, which are reflected in their more diffuse neural networks, spanning subcortical nuclei that connect with the cortex via the white matter.

At this point, a closer look at the functional role of the cerebral white matter is called for. Although Cummings and Benson (1984) have stressed that subcortical dementia is a clinical, not an anatomical concept, focusing exclusively on the deep grey matter effectively ignored almost 50% of the total cerebral volume. The functional importance of the cerebral white matter is well illustrated in a brief description of the neural circuitry subserving attention. Attention, may be defined as a subject's ability to attend to a specific stimulus without being distracted by extraneous environmental stimuli (Strub and Black, 1977), and impairment in this basic aspect of cognition, is one of the hallmarks of demyelinating disease (Filley et al., 1989a; Feinstein et al., 1993; Kujala et al., 1995). Mesulam (1981) has identified four distinct contributions (sensory, motor, limbic and reticular activation) to the overall organization of one aspect of attention, namely spatially directed attention. All are richly interconnected. Spatially directed attention is thus a balance between ascending (reticular–cortical) activation and cortical (cortico-reticular) modulation, the limbic system adding emotional importance to the object of attention and conscious voluntary effort supplied by the frontal lobes. A pivotal cortical area integrating sensory input is the dorsolateral portion of the posterior parietal cortex. This area contains an elaborate sensory representation of extrapersonal space, a prerequisite for distributing attention. The frontal cortex, particularly the frontal eye fields and surrounding regions, assist in initiating or inhibiting motor mechanisms involved in attentive behaviour. Damage to this area manifests as failure to orientate, manipulate and explore perceptual representations. The anatomical separation of sensory and motor components is not, however, complete. Some sensory representation occurs in the frontal cortex and vice versa, an arrangement shown to improve functional efficiency (Mesulam, 1981). The cingulate region, with extensive limbic connections, gives motivational relevance to sensory events which may then receive more extensive representation in the dorsolateral parietal cortex, thereby enhancing activation of frontal mechanisms. Finally, an intact reticular formation is essential in maintaining arousal, without which attention and vigilance becomes impaired.

For object specific attention, additional components are required, e.g. association areas in regions such as the inferior temporal cortex are concerned with features of an object such as colour, texture and shape (Wise and Demisone, 1988).

A single lesion occurring anywhere within this extensive network may therefore disrupt functional integrity through a process of disconnection (Geschwind, 1965). The same holds for any of the myriad neural networks underpinning every aspect of behaviour, and the cerebral white matter is particularly important in this regard, for it fulfils an essential integrative function, reciprocally linking cortical to other cortical and subcortical areas. It has long been recognized that a brain lesion may produce disordered cerebral function at another site, a process termed diaschisis. In conditions that diffusely affect the white matter, such as multiple sclerosis, the concept has been demonstrated through a combination of structural (CT) and functional (PET) neuroimaging (Brooks et al., 1984) with primarily white matter lesions producing a global reduction in cortical cerebral perfusion.

White matter neurobehavioural syndromes

In trying to ascertain whether there is a specific behavioural syndrome pertinent to white matter pathology, the researcher confronts the same dilemmas that first confronted those defining the behavioural characteristics of the basal ganglia disorders in the 1970s. During the intervening years, improved technology has demonstrated, in vivo, that to understand cerebral function is to understand the role of neural networks. With neural networks spanning the cortical, subcortical grey and white matter, it is even more relevant today to repeat Cummings and Benson's (1984) assertion that the term subcortical should be regarded more as a clinical than an anatomical approbation. But, even this cautionary note is somewhat disingenuous, for the cerebral white matter is a distinct anatomical entity. Although inextricably linked to cortical and subcortical areas, the unique anatomical and physiological properties of white matter suggest that pathology confined to it may have a distinct clinical profile. This raises the question of whether there are conditions that exclusively target the cerebral white matter? Disorders such as MS, considered a prototypical white matter disease, do not totally spare the cortex, and the same could be said for other conditions be they

Table 10.1 Adult cerebral white matter disorders

Demyelinating	Multiple Sclerosis
Vascular	Binswanger's disease
	Stroke
Toxic	Alcoholic dementia
	Toluene dementia
	Radiation
	Chemotherapy
Infectious	Acquired immune deficiency syndrome
	Progressive multifocal leukoencephalopathy
Metabolic	Hypoxia
	Cobalamin deficiency
	Marchiafava Bignami disease
	Central pontine myelinosis
Traumatic	Traumatic brain injury
	Corpus callosotomy
Neoplastic	Tumours
	Gliomatosis cerebri

vascular, toxic or infective. In referring to the various conditions below as white matter disorders, the assumption is that they predominantly, but not exclusively, involve the cerebral white matter.

Disorders of the cerebral white matter

A comprehensive list of disorders affecting the cerebral white matter has been provided by Filley (1996) (Table 10.1), who has noted the paucity of associated neurobehavioural data compared with cortically based conditions. A distinction is made between adult and childhood disorders, although it is recognized that some conditions may apply to both age groups. The childhood disorders will not be considered here, the exception being metachromatic leukodystrophy.

Most of the neurobehavioural research in this area has been undertaken in patients with MS, regarded as the prototypical white matter disease. Taking MS as a central reference point with which to compare results from other conditions, a MEDLINE search going back 10 years was undertaken, looking for neuropsychiatric studies that compared MS with either (a) white matter disorders, (b) deep grey matter disorders and (c) cortical disorders. The yield was small. With respect to the white matter, two studies comparing MS to the Acquired Immunodeficiency Syndrome (AIDS) and Traumatic Brain Injury (TBI) respectively, were found. Given these comparisons and the fact that both AIDS and TBI are amongst the most frequently encountered subcortical white matter diseases, more detailed clinicopathological descriptions of them are provided. In addition, two other white matter disorders will be discussed in greater detail as they have been the focus of research interest; Binswanger's disease as an example of the etiological and clinical uncertainty surrounding aspects of vascular dementia and metachromatic leukodystrophy because of the strong association with psychosis. Finally, neuropsychological studies comparing MS with cortical (Alzheimer's disease) and subcortical grey matter (Huntington's disease) are discussed, and the section concludes with some comments on recovery of function.

Acquired immune deficiency syndrome

The acquired immune deficiency syndrome (AIDS) results from infection with the human immunodeficiency virus (HIV). Neuropsychiatric sequelae may result from the direct effect of HIV on the CNS, or the many secondary diseases associated with the AIDS syndrome. The term Aids Dementia Complex was put forward by physicians to describe changes in mentation and motor function that were not attributable to CNS tumours, opportunistic infections and systemic diseases (Navia et al. 1986). AIDS has been regarded as primarily a subcortical disease because the virus has a predilection for the central white matter and deep grey structures, such as the basal ganglia, thalamus and brainstem, leaving the cortex relatively unaffected. White et al. (1995) have reviewed the literature from 57 studies that compared the presence or absence of cognitive deficits in asymptomatic HIV seropositive and seronegative subjects. The median rate of neuropsychological impairment for the seropositive group was 35%, compared with 12% for the seronegative group. Thus, changes in mentation may precede physical signs and symptoms of HIV infection and the reported symptoms of slowing, learning efficiency, apathy and avoidance of complex tasks (Markowitz and Perry, 1992) suggest a subcortical dementing process. There is also evidence that cognitive impairment may increase as the disease progresses with deficits attributable to cerebral involvement (mainly white matter atrophy), rather than associated mood changes, substance abuse or constitutional symptoms (Heaton et al., 1995).

The typical MRI picture is one of diffuse white matter high signal lesions (Olsen et al., 1988)(Fig. 10.1), and lesion detection may be improved with the use of contrast enhancement (Tuite et al., 1993). Multifocal, as opposed to diffuse white matter lesions, are more typical of progressive multifocal leukoencephalopathy, a papova virus infection that may occur together with AIDS (Fig. 10.2).

Traumatic brain injury

Over three million people in the United States suffer a traumatic brain injury each year (Collins, 1990), making it by far the most frequent cause of acquired brain injury. While evidence of cortical damage may be readily

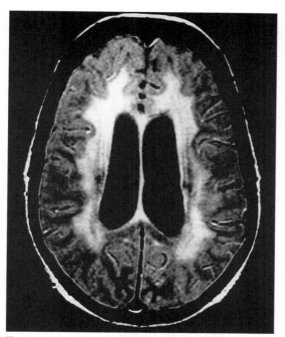

Fig. 10.1   An axial proton density (spin echo) MRI in a 25-year-old male with HIV dementia. The CSF appears hypointense and offsets the extensive periventricular, confluent white matter lesions.

discernable, often to the naked eye (e.g. subdural and intracerebral bleeds) it is now also recognized that the cerebral white matter may be adversely affected. Extensive white matter degeneration was noted by Strich (1961) at postmortem in patients who had survived for months in a comatose state. She proposed that lesions resulted from a direct tearing of nerve fibres at the time of impact, although others argued they were secondary to raised intracranial pressure (Jellinger and Seitelberg, 1970). The argument has been resolved, as it is now accepted that diffuse axonal injury, affecting the cerebral white matter, can occur following a closed (non-penetrating) head injury, in the absence of raised intracranial pressure (Adams et al., 1977).

In vivo evidence of cerebral involvement has come for neuroimaging and neuropsychological studies of patients with moderate to mild closed head injuries. Levin et al. (1987) showed that at least 80% of patients had cerebral lesions visible on CT or MRI within days of sustaining the injury. The majority of lesions were localized to frontal and temporal regions and were associated with neuropsychological deficits pertaining to frontal lobe and memory tasks. Of the 39 parenchymal lesions demonstrated by MRI, 27 involved both the grey and white matter, while fewer were confined either to the white or grey matter alone. Serial MRI follow-up of a similar sample

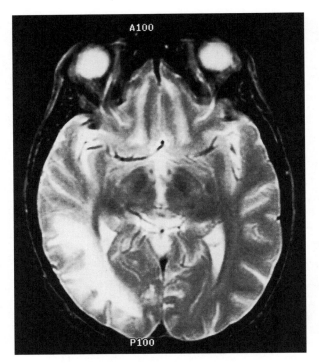

Fig. 10.2   An axial T_2-weighted (spin echo) MRI in a 27-year-old male with progressive multifocal leukoencephalopathy.

(Levin et al., 1992) demonstrated substantial lesion resolution by 3 months, with a concomitant improvement in neuropsychological deficits. Nevertheless, some patients whose lesions had resolved by 1 month continued to perform poorly on tests of executive function and memory. The reason for this was provided by functional neuroimaging (positron emission tomography), which demonstrated reduced glucose metabolism in brain regions deemed normal on structural neuroimaging (Humayun et al., 1989; Ruff et al., 1994), abnormalities correlating with deficits in attention and memory. Significantly, some of the patients with neuropsychological and PET deficits had not lost consciousness, but rather had experienced an alteration in consciousness at the time of injury, demonstrating that mild TBI may, in some cases, lead to demonstrable deficits in cerebral function.

Vascular: Binswanger's disease

Binswanger's disease has also been termed subcortical arteriosclerotic encephalopathy (Babikian and Ropper, 1987) and is thought to arise from chronic cerebral ischemia, primarily affecting the white matter. Hypertension is frequently implicated (Babikian and Ropper, 1987), cerebral amyloid angiopathy less so (Gray et al., 1985), but the precise pathogenesis is unclear. Similarly, the relationship of the disorder to white matter lesions viewed on MRI in asymptomatic elderly (Filley et al., 1989b) or middle-aged subjects (Rao et al., 1989) is open to debate (see Chapter 9). The confluent, periventricular white matter lesions seen on T_2-weighted MRI may be indistinguishable from MS (Fig. 10.3) and the clinical presentation compatible with that of subcortical dementia. Although Binswanger's disease is considered a separate clinical entity from other vascular causes of dementia such as multi-infarct dementia and stroke, more recently recognized causes of vascular mediated white matter change, such as the genetic variant, cerebral autosomal dominant arteriopathy with subcortical infarcts and leukoencephalopathy (CADASIL) (Stevens et al., 1977; Salloway, 1996) should also be part of any differential diagnosis.

Metachromatic leukodystrophy (MLD)
First described by Alzheimer (1910), this familial disease with an autosomal recessive mode of inheritance, is caused by a deficiency or absence in the enzyme arylsulfatase A. An accumulation of sulphatides ensues in the nervous system which causes demyelination of axons and peripheral nerves. The age of presentation, which may vary from infancy to adulthood, is dependent on the degree of enzyme deficiency, the less severe the later the onset (Polten et al., 1991). Neuroimaging reveals that demyelination in MLD usually starts in the frontal lobes affecting the periventricular white matter and corpus callosum, before spreading more posteriorly.

A feature of the adolescent and early adult onset MLD is the high prevalence of psychosis, estimated to be in excess of 50% (Hyde et al., 1992). The clinical presentation is frequently indistinguishable from schizophrenia, with patients displaying prominent and bizarre delusions and hallucinations. The occurrence of psychosis is age-related, giving way to dementia as the patient gets older. Thus, psychosis appears dependent on intact, albeit pathologically, functioning neural circuitry, which is predominantly located in frontal white matter. With the progression of demyelination, frontal subcortical circuits are presumably ablated with a subsequent resolution of psychosis.

What is intriguing about MLD is that the disorder, which primarily affects the white matter, is associated with such a high prevalence of psychosis, a condition firmly associated with cortical involvement. Hyde et al. (1992), in their comprehensive review of all published reports of MLD have concluded that the prevalence of psychosis far exceeds other neurological disorders that are also linked to psychosis, such as temporal lobe epilepsy (Roberts et al., 1990) and Huntington's disease (Dewhurst et al., 1969). The implications of this finding are that white matter tracts, particularly those connected to the frontal lobes, play a pivotal role in the pathogenesis of psychosis, presumably by disconnecting the frontal cortex from other important loci implicated in

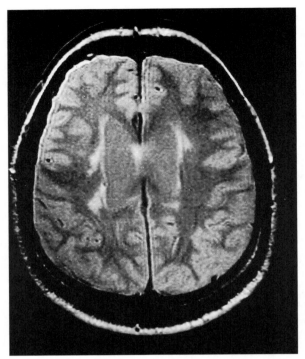

Fig. 10.3 An axial MRI (proton density, spin echo sequence) in a 44-year-old male with Binswanger's subcortical encephalopathy, demonstrating periventricular confluent white matter lesions.

psychosis, such as the medial temporal lobe, basal ganglia and diencephalon (Davison and Bagley, 1969). Psychosis should thus no longer be regarded as the preserve of cortical pathology (Filley and Gross, 1992) and, like cognition, is best conceptualized as an age-related phenomenon, dependent, amongst other things, on the integrity of the subcortical frontal white matter. The temporal sequence of events in MLD needs to be emphasized, because other white matter diseases such as MS are infrequently associated with psychosis. The different pattern and extent of lesion distribution in MS may also account for this observation.

Neurobehavioural comparisons between MS and cortical, deep grey matter and white matter disorders

Comparisons of this nature are beset by methodological difficulties. Controlling for different demographic features and varying degrees of cerebral involvement, disability, disease severity and disease course will always be, at best, an imprecise exercise. Thus, in interpreting the findings, considerable caution should be adopted. Nevertheless, looking for similarities and differences according to the anatomical substrate affected makes intuitive sense, for this method allows the researcher to test a priori assumptions with respect to descriptive and, to some extent, construct validity.

MS and acquired immunodeficiency disease

A comparison between three groups of 20 patients each, namely MS, AIDS and HIV seronegative subjects (the latter used as a control group), illustrates some of the hazards mentioned above (Morriss et al., 1992). The AIDS subjects were homosexual males and, to achieve a demographic match, the MS sample was limited to males as well, an atypical situation in a disorder with a female preponderance. In addition, the MS sample was significantly older than the other two groups, which was controlled for using analysis of covariance, a method considered problematic when dealing with demographic mismatch (Adams et al, 1985).

The cognitive findings demonstrated a three-way split in that AIDS patients occupied an intermediate position between the MS and HIV seronegative group. MS patients were more likely to show cognitive impairment, but when the demographic confounders were eliminated, this difference was only apparent for performance on the Symbol Digit Modalities Test (SDMT). Regarding psychopathology, the MS patients were significantly more likely to develop an affective disorder following the onset of their neurological symptoms, whereas the AIDS group described more premorbid mental illness and more current mental illness (anxiety disorders, psychosis, adjustment disorders) with the exception of affective disorder. Although the authors concluded major differences in mentation were present between MS and AIDS patients, a contrary interpretation can be suggested. The limited psychometric battery concentrated on speed of information processing, verbal fluency and some indices of motor sequencing (Luria three-step procedure; go no-go tests). Performances between MS and AIDS patients were similar on all measures except the SDMT although, even here, AIDS patients performed more poorly than their matched HIV seronegative control group, indicating they too had difficulties with attention and processing speed. As for the psychiatric differences, these are hard to interpret because of biased sample selection. Viewed from this perspective, the study offers some tentative evidence of overlap, at least in the cognitive domain, between two common causes of white matter pathology. Larger, more representative sample selection and an expanded psychometric battery are needed before more definite conclusions can be reached.

MS and Traumatic Brain Injury

Having made the case earlier that TBI represents one of the commonest causes of white matter damage and that changes in cognition are consonant with features of subcortical dementia, the only study to directly compare neuropsychological abnormalities in MS and TBI failed to demonstrate common areas of deficit (Horton and Siegel, 1990). Instead, the profile to emerge in the TBI patients was one of cortical deficits which contrasted with the deficits noted in the MS patients. However, the very small sample size, limited psychometric battery and the absence of any data describing the type or site of the TBI effectively negates the significance of the results. The study is nevertheless cited because it is a good example of the problems that may arise when comparing different disorders.

MS and Alzheimer's disease

Many studies have upheld the cortical–subcortical behavioural dichotomy by directly comparing the neuropsychological profiles of patients with Alzheimer's disease on the one hand and those with Huntington's disease (Brandt et al., 1988; Salmon et al., 1989; Troster et al., 1989; Rouleau et al., 1992; Paulsen et al., 1995) and Parkinson's disease (Pillon et al., 1991; Bancher et al., 1993), on the other. Only a single study has, however, contrasted the cognitive performances of Alzheimer and MS patients (Filley et al., 1989c). Controlling for the effects of age, sex and education mismatch, the Alzheimer patients were found to be more globally demented and, when in turn this was controlled for, greater deficits in verbal skills, memory, learning and visuo-spatial function were noted. MS patients were relatively more impaired on psychomotor tasks, and particular emphasis was placed on disturbances in attention as a principal mental state abnormality in MS. The results supported a distinct subcortical cognitive profile, but the authors acknowledged the heterogenous nature of subcortical brain pathology and suggested a further subdivision into white and grey matter dementias. However, this would have required the demonstration of neurobehavioural differences between white matter and basal ganglia disorders, something beyond the scope of Filley et al.'s study.

MS and Huntington's disease

Neuropsychological investigation revealed that the overall pattern of deficits in MS patients was similar to those seen in Huntington's disease (HD), although some individual differences were still discernable (Caine et al., 1986). The study was methodologically robust because globally demented patients and those on psychoactive medication were excluded, a comprehensive battery of tests utilised and attempts made to match the groups with respect to functional disability. In addition, the inclusion of a normal control group illustrated that although MS patients were less impaired than the HD group, in relation to healthy subjects, both subcortical diseases were associated with widespread cognitive deficits.

The differences between the patient groups could be summarized as follows: language difficulties, visuospatial (copying) deficits and dyscalculia were more prominent in the HD subjects. While both HD and MS patients showed memory deficits, these were more marked in the HD patients who had problems both with retrieval and verbal recognition. MS patients did relatively well on verbal recognition tasks and their difficulties were largely confined to those of retrieval. The latter could explain the mild naming deficits noted in MS patients, which occurred in the absence of other language abnormalities. Speed of cognition in MS was noted to be slow.

The study was important for a number of reasons. Coming at a time of renewed interest in the concept of subcortical dementia (Cummings and Benson, 1984; Cummings, 1986; Rao, 1986), the similar overall pattern of cognitive deficits in two disorders regarded as quintessentially subcortical, added support to the notion of a different kind of dementia. But, the study went further and, by demonstrating cortical (language) deficits in subcortical disorders (HD), also showed that the two areas were not functionally independent. Caine and colleagues were also the first to delineate the more subtle cognitive differences that characterize white matter and subcortical grey matter disease, thereby adding impetus not only to the notion of a subcortical dementia, but more specifically, to a subcortical white matter dementia.

A final point to note is that neither of the studies comparing MS patients to those with HD (Caine et al., 1986) or Alzheimer's disease (Filley et al. 1989c) made mention of implicit (procedural) memory. This refers to motor skills (driving, playing a musical instrument), classical conditioning and priming. HD patients show deficits in motor skill learning (Heindel et al., 1988), but have intact priming (Shinamura et al., 1987), whereas Alzheimer patients have the reverse, i.e. difficulty with priming tasks (Salmon et al., 1988), but intact motor learning skills (Heindel et al., 1988). MS patients do not have problems with either priming (Beatty and Monson, 1990) or motor learning skills (Beatty et al., 1990), thus suggesting a further discriminating cognitive feature.

Recovery of function

There is evidence that the cerebral white, but not grey, matter may show varying degrees of recovery from insult. Serial MRI has demonstrated the waxing and waning of white matter plaques (Miller et al., 1988) and improvement in mentation may follow suite (Rozewicz et al., 1996). The ability of myelin to spontaneously regenerate, although limited, has been pursued as a possible treatment option in disorders such as MS (ffrench-Constant, 1994). Many possible treatment options for an array of white matter disorders have been reviewed by Filley (1996), and range from surgical correction of normal pressure hydrocephalus to the potential reversibility of cognitive decline in abstinent alcoholics. Irrespective of the disorder, similar recovery is not possible after cortical destruction.

Summary

- Multiple sclerosis as a demyelinating disease, predominantly affects the white matter. Given that the cortex is less frequently involved, cognitive dysfunction associated with MS may be termed a subcortical dementia.
- The hallmarks of a subcortical dementia are forgetfulness, a slowness of thought processes, emotional or personality changes (summarized as apathy or depression interspersed with irritability), and an impaired ability to manipulate acquired knowledge.
- Aphasia, apraxia, and agnosia, all characteristic of a cortical dementia, are not found in patients with a subcortical dementing process.
- The early descriptions of subcortical dementia were limited to patients with basal ganglia disease, which begs the question to what degree do the neurobehavioural aspects of MS differ from these disorders ?
- Unlike the basal ganglia disorders, MS is not associated with movement disorders nor deficits in implicit memory. There are also qualitative differences in explicit memory deficits.
- There is evidence that the cerebral white matter, unlike the grey, may show varying degrees of recovery from insult, thereby establishing another important difference between these two substrates.
- However, descriptive validity for a distinct 'subcortical, white matter dementia' still needs to be established. To do this, neurobehavioural comparisons between MS and other predominantly white matter diseases such as HIV dementia, metachromatic leukodystrophy and Binswanger's subcortical encephalopathy, need to be undertaken.

References

Adams KM, Brown GG, Grant I. (1985) Analysis of covariance as a remedy for demographic mismatch of research subject groups: some sobering simulations. *Journal of Clinical and Experimental Neuropsychology*, **7**, 445–62.

Adams JH, Mitchell DE, Graham DI, Doyle D. (1977) Diffuse brain damage of immediate impact type. *Brain*, **100**, 489–502.

Albert ML. (1978) Subcortical dementia. In *Alzheimer's Disease: Senile Dementia and Related Disorders*, ed. R Katzman, RD Terry, KL Bick. New York: Raven Press.

Albert ML, Feldman RG, Willis AL. (1974) The 'subcortical dementia' of progressive supranuclear palsy. *Journal of Neurology, Neurosurgery and Psychiatry*, **37**, 121–30.

Alexander GE, Crutcher MD. (1990) Functional architecture of basal ganglia circuits: neural substrates of parallel processing. *Trends in Neuroscience*, **13**, 266–71.

Alexander GE, DeLong MR, Strick PL. (1986) Parallel organisation of functionally segregated circuits linking basal ganglia and cortex. *Annual Review of Neuroscience*, **9**, 357–81.

Alzheimer A. (1910) Beitrag zur Kenntnis der pathologischen Neuroglis und ihrer Beziehungen zu Abbauvorgangen Nervengewebe. In *Histologische und histopathologische Arbeiten uber die Grosshirnrinde*, ed. F Nissl, A Alzheimer. pp. 401–4. Jena, Federal Republic of Germany: Gustav Fischer.

American Psychiatric Association. (1994) *The Diagnostic and Statistical Manual of Mental Disorders*, Fourth Edition. Washington, DC: American Psychiatric Association.

Babikian V, Ropper AH. (1987) Binswanger's disease: a review. *Stroke*, **18**, 2–12.

Bancher C, Braak H, Fischer P, Jellinger KA. (1993) Neuropsychological staging of Alzheimer lesions and intellectual, status in Alzheimer's and Parkinson's disease patients. *Neuroscience Letters*, **162**, 179–82.

Beatty WW, Monson N. (1990) Semantic priming in multiple sclerosis. *Bulletin of the Psychonomic Society*, **28**, 397–400.

Beatty WW, Goodkin DE, Monson N, Beatty PA. (1990) Implicit learning in patients with chronic-progressive multiple sclerosis. *International Journal of Clinical Neuropsychology*, **12**, 166–72.

Brandt J, Folstein SE, Folstein MF. (1988) Differential cognitive impairment in Alzheimer's disease and Huntington's disease. *Annals of Neurology*, **23**, 555–61.

Brooks DJ, Leenders KL, Head G, Marshall J, Legg NJ et al. (1984) Studies on regional cerebral oxygen utilisation and cognitive function in multiple sclerosis. *Journal of Neurology, Neurosurgery and Psychiatry*, **47**, 1182–91.

Caine ED, Shoulson I.(1983) Psychiatric syndromes in Huntington's disease. *American Journal of Psychiatry*, **140**, 728–33.

Caine ED, Bamford KA, Schiffer RB, Shoulson I, Levy S. (1986) A controlled neuropsychological comparison of Huntington's disease and multiple sclerosis. *Archives of Neurology*, **43**, 249–54.

Collins JG. (1990) Types of injuries by selected characteristics: United States, 1985–1987. *Vital and Health Statistics, Series 10: Data from the National Health Survey, No. 175. DHHS Publication No [PHS]91–1503*. Hyattsville, MD: US Department of Health and Human Services.

Cummings JL. (1986) Subcortical dementia. Neuropsychology, neuropsychiatry, and pathophysiology. *British Journal of Psychiatry*, **149**, 682–97.

Cummings JL. (1993) Frontal-subcortical circuits and human behaviour. *Archives of Neurology*, **50**, 873–80.

Cummings JL, Benson F. (1984) Subcortical dementia. Review of an emerging concept. *Archives of Neurology*, **41**, 874–9.

Davison K, Bagley CR. (1969) Schizophrenia-like psychoses associated with organic disorders of the central nervous system: a review of the literature. In *Current Problems in Neuropsychiatry*, ed. RN Harrington, pp. 113–84. Ashford, Kent: Headley.

Dewhurst K, Oliver J, Trick KLK, McKnight AL. (1969) Neuropsychiatric aspects of

Huntington's disease. *Confina Neurologica*, **31**, 258–68.

Feinstein A, Ron MA. (1990) Psychosis associated with demonstrable brain disease. *Psychological Medicine*, **20**, 793–803.

Feinstein A, Ron MA, Thompson A. (1993) A serial study of psychometric and magnetic resonance imaging changes in multiple sclerosis. *Brain*, **116**, 569–602.

ffrench-Constant C. (1994) Pathogenesis of multiple sclerosis. *Lancet*, **343**, 271–4.

Filley CM. (1996) Neurobehavioural aspects of cerebral white matter disorders. In *Neuropsychiatry*, ed. BS Fogel, RB Schiffer. pp. 913–34. Baltimore: Williams and Wilkins.

Filley CM, Gross KF. (1992) Psychosis with cerebral white matter. *Neuropsychiatry, Neuropsychology and Behavioural Neurology*, **5**, 119–25.

Filley CM, Davis KA, Schmitz SP et al. (1989b) Neuropsychological performance and magnetic resonance imaging in Alzheimer's disease and normal aging. *Neuropsychiatry, Neuropsychology, and Behavioural Neurology*, **2**, 81–91.

Filley CM, Franklin GM, Heaton RK, Rodenberg NL. (1989a) White matter dementia. Clinical disorders and implications. *Neuropsychiatry, Neuropsychology and Behavioural Neurology*, **1**, 239–54.

Filley CM, Heaton RK, Nelson LM, Burks JS, Franklin GM. (1989c) A comparison of dementia in Alzheimer's disease and multiple sclerosis. *Archives of Neurology*, **46**, 157–61.

Geschwind N. (1965) Disconnection syndromes in animals and man. *Brain*, **88**, 237–94.

Gray F, Dubas F, Roullet E, Escourolle R. (1985) Leukoencephalopathy in diffuse haemorrhagic cerebral amyloid angiopathy. *Annals of Neurology*, **18**, 54–9.

Hakim AM, Mathieson G. (1979) Dementia in Parkinson's disease. A neuropathologic study. *Neurology*, **29**, 1209–14.

Harvey I, Ron MA, du Boulay GE, Wicks D, Lewis SW, Murray RM. (1993) Reduction in cortical volume in schizophrenia on magnetic resonance imaging. *Psychological Medicine*, **23**, 591–604.

Heaton RK, Grant I, Butters N, White DA.(1995) The HNRC 500: neuropsychology of HIV infection at different disease stages. *The Journal of the International Neuropsychological Society*, **1**, 231–51.

Heindel WC, Butters N, Salmon DP. (1988) Impaired learning of a motor skill in patients with Huntington's disease. *Behavioural Neuroscience*, **102**, 141–7.

Horton AM, Siegel E. (1990) Comparison of multiple sclerosis and head trauma patients: a neuropsychological pilot study. *International Journal of Neuroscience*, **53**, 213–15.

Humayun MS, Presty SK, Lafrance ND et al. (1989) Local cerebral glucose abnormalities in mild closed head injured patients with cognitive impairment. *Nuclear Medicine Communications*, **10**, 335–44.

Hyde TM, Ziegler JC, Weinberger DR. (1992) Psychiatric disturbances in metachromatic leukodystrophy. Insights in to the neurobiology of psychosis. *Archives of Neurology*, **49**, 401–6.

Jellinger K, Seitelberg G. (1970) Protracted post-traumatic encephalopathy: pathology, pathogenesis and clinical implications. *Journal of Neurological Sciences*, **10**, 51–94.

Johansson B, Roos B-E. (1974) 5–Hydroxyindoleacetic acid and homovanillic acid in cerebrospinal fluid of patients with neurological disease. *European Neurology*, 11, 37–45.

Kujala P, Portin R, Revonsuo A, Ruutiainen J. (1995) Attention related performance in two cognitively different subgroups of patients with multiple sclerosis. *Journal of Neurology, Neurosurgery and Psychiatry*, 59, 77–82.

Levin HS, Amparo E, Eisenberg HM et al. (1987) Magnetic resonance imaging and computerised tomography in relation to the neurobehavioural sequelae of mild and moderate head injuries. *Journal of Neurosurgery*, 66, 706–13.

Levin HS, Williams DH, Eisenberg HM, High WM, Guinto FC. (1992) Serial MRI and neurobehavioural findings after mild to moderate closed head injury. *Journal of Neurology, Neurosurgery and Psychiatry*, 55, 255–62.

Markowitz JC, Perry SW. (1992) Effects of the Human Immunodeficiency Virus on the central nervous system. In *Textbook of Neuropsychiatry*, ed. SC Yudowsky, RE Hales. ch. 21. pp. 499–518. Washington DC: American Psychiatric Press.

Markianos M, Sfagos C. (1988) Altered serotonin uptake kinetics in multiple sclerosis. *Journal of Neurology*, 235, 236–7.

McHugh PR, Folstein MF. (1975) Psychiatric syndromes of Huntington's chorea: a clinical and phenomenologic study. In *Psychiatric Aspects of Neurologic Disease*, ed. DF Benson, D Blumer. New York: Grune and Stratton.

Mesulam M-M. (1981) Large scale neurocognitive networks and distributed processing for attention, language and memory. *Annals of Neurology*, 28, 597–613.

Miller DH, Rudge P, Johnson G, Kendall BE, MacManus DG, Moseley IF, McDonald WI. (1988) Serial gadolinium enhanced MRI in multiple sclerosis. *Brain*, 111, 927–39.

Monsch AU, Bondi MW, Butters N et al. (1994) A comparison of category and letter fluency in Alzheimer's disease and Huntington's disease. *Neuropsychology*, 8, 25–30.

Morriss R, Schaerf F, Brandt J, McArthur J, Folstein M. (1992) AIDS and multiple sclerosis: neural and mental features. *Acta Psychiatrica Scandinavica*, 85, 331–6.

Navia BA, Jordan BD, Price RW. (1986) The AIDS dementia complex, I: clinical features. *Annals of Neurology*, 19, 517–24.

Olsen WL, Longo FM, Mills CM, Norman D. (1988) White matter disease in AIDS: findings at MR imaging. *Neuroradiology*, 169, 445–8.

Paulsen JS, Butters N, Sadek JR et al. (1995) Distinct cognitive profiles of cortical and subcortical dementia in advanced illness. *Neurology*, 45, 951–6.

Pillon B, Dubois B, Ploska A, Agid Y. (1991) Severity and specificity of cognitive impairment in Alzheimer's, Huntington's, and Parkinson's diseases and progressive supranuclear palsy. *Neurology*, 41, 634–43.

Polten A, Fluharty AL, Fluharty CB, Kappler J, von Figura K, Gieselmann V. (1991) Molecular basis of different forms of metachromatic leukodystrophy. *New England Journal of Medicine*, 324, 18–22.

Rao SM. (1986) Neuropsychology of multiple sclerosis: a critical review. *Journal of Clinical and Experimental Neuropsychology*, 8, 503–42.

Rao SM, Mittenberg W, Bernardin L, Haughton V, Leo GJ. (1989) Neuropsychological test findings in subjects with leukoaraiosis. *Archives of Neurology*, 46, 40–4.

Roberts GW, Done DJ, Bruton C, Crow TJ. (1990). A 'mock-up' of schizophrenia: temporal lobe epilepsy and schizophrenia-like psychoses. *Biological Psychiatry*. 28,

127–43.

Rouleau I, Salmon DP, Butters N, Kennedy C, McGuire K. (1992) Quantitative and qualitative analyses of clock drawings in Alzheimer's and Huntington's disease. *Brain and Cognition*, **18**, 70–87.

Rozewicz L, Langdon DW, Davie CA, Thompson AJ, Ron MA. (1996) Resolution of left hemisphere cognitive dysfunction in multiple sclerosis with magnetic resonance correlates: a case report. *Cognitive Neuropsychiatry*, **1**, 17–25.

Ruff RM, Crouch JA, Troster AI et al. (1994) Selected cases of poor outcome following minor brain trauma: comparing neuropsychological and positron emission tomography assessment. *Brain Injury*, **8**, 297–308.

Salloway S. (1996) Clinico-pathologic case conference: depression, behaviour change and subcortical dementia in a 57 year old woman. *Journal of Neuropsychiatry and Clinical Neurosciences*, **8**, 215–21.

Salmon DP, Kwo-on-Yen PF, Heindel WC, Butters N, Thal LJ. (1989) Differentiation of Alzheimer's disease and Huntington's disease with the dementia rating scale. *Archives of Neurology*, **46**, 1204–8.

Salmon DP, Shinamura AP, Butters N, Smith S. (1988) Lexical and semantic priming deficits in patients with Alzheimer's disease. *Journal of Clinical and Experimental Neuropsychology*, **10**, 477–94.

Shinamura AP, Salmon DP, Squire LR, Butters N. (1987) Memory dysfunction and word priming in dementia and amnesia. *Behavioural Neuroscience*, **101**, 347–51.

Stevens, DL, Hewlett RH, Brownell B. (1977) Chronic-familial vascular encephalopathy. *Lancet*, **i**, 1364–5.

Strich SJ. (1961) Shearing of nerve fibres as a cause of brain damage due to head injury. *Lancet*, **ii**, 443–68.

Strub RL, Black FW. (1977) The mental status examination in neurology. Philadelphia: FA Davis Co.

Suddath RL, Christison GW, Torrey EF. (1990) Anatomical abnormalities in the brains of monozygotic twins discordant for schizophrenia. *New England Journal of Medicine*, **322**, 789–94.

Troster AI, Salmon DP, McCullough D, Butters N. (1989) A comparison of the category fluency deficits associated with Alzheimer's and Huntington's disease. *Brain and Language*, **37**, 500–13.

Tuite M, Ketonenen L, Kieburtz K, Handy B. (1993) Efficacy of gadolinium in MR brain imaging of HIV-infected patients. *American Journal of Neuroradiology*, **14**, 257–63.

White DA, Heaton RK, Monsch AU, and the HNRC Group. (1995) Neuropsychological studies of asymptomatic Human Immunodeficiency Virus-Type-1 infected individuals. *Journal of the International Neuropsychological Society*, **1**, 304–15.

Whitehouse PJ, Price DL, Struble RG, Clark AW, Coyle JT, DeLong MR. (1982) Alzheimer's disease and senile dementia: loss of neurons in the basal forebrain. *Science*, **215**, 1237–9.

Wilson SAK. (1912) Progressive lenticular degeneration: a familial nervous disease associated with cirrhosis of the liver. *Brain*, **34**, 295–509.

Wise SP, Demisone R. (1988) Behavioural neurophysiology: insights into seeing and grasping. *Science*, **242**, 736–41.

Index